MOVEMENT IS BLISS

This is What Matters Most When You Move

by Suresha Hill, EdS, HSE, DOMTP

Somatic Intelligence – Volume 9

MOVEMENT IS BLISS

This Is What Matters Most When You Move

Simple sequences that release tension, awaken deadened cells, and revitalize your relationship with your body

Written by

Suresha Hill, EdS, HSE, DOMTP

(Educational Specialist, Hanna Somatic Educator, Diplomate in Osteopathic Manipulative Theory and Practice)

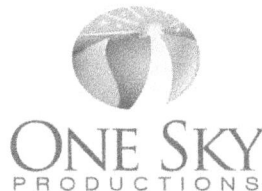

ONE SKY
PRODUCTIONS

TABLE OF CONTENTS

Disclaimer

Although the explorations and movement sequences are gentle and intended to awaken and reset the body into greater and greater degrees of balance and integration, the way they are carried out can neither be monitored nor corrected using this format.

They are not intended to replace medical advice or treatments. Consult your doctor before attempting to assume any of the recommended postures if you feel there is any possibility of harm to a fragile system or condition.

Numerous movements described involve changing joint position in relation to other areas of the body, and they are designed to increase mobility and balance. But be mindful if you have had surgeries or injuries; damaged or degenerative discs; tears in the joint capsule or rotator cuff muscles, ligaments, tendons or knees; or sprains that have created restrictive scar tissue.

Any of these scenarios can potentially be greatly improved by somatic movements and manual methods if done slowly, gradually, gently, and consciously, but you must assume responsibility to monitor your own body's tolerance and responsiveness moment to moment.

Acknowledgments

I've already mentioned the specific names of people who were most influential in the career path that opened up, in every other Volume, but the culmination of influences for this book needs a wider acknowledgment. The best way to sum up the contributors to the information in this book that stems from a combination of experience and study, contemplation and meditation, is to honor Life as the best ever teacher.

Life has been the overarching manifestation of synchronistic circumstances, people, and even accidents and injuries that have been transformative. Life has brought them all in such a perfect sequence that at times it even felt magical in the timing of the steps that were presented to be climbed. I will be forever grateful for the solutions that arose and for the questions that sparked them. Life listens and sends the right teachers, like Dr. Tom Hanna, without whom this chapter In my life would not have happened.

The graphics were chosen to reflect their alignment with Nature, the mystery, exquisite architecture, and fluid geometry of the body, as well as it being a sacred site to hold all that life brings with infinite capacity to transduce and transmit both from them and from us in the process.

> *"The "I AM" consciousness is love, bliss. Out of bliss of parents' union the I is born. All consciousness is chemical and everything is mechanical. It just happens spontaneously. The basis or screen upon which it happens is the Absolute."*
>
> *Nisargadatta Maharaj*

(Image courtesy of Diego F. Parra and Pexels)

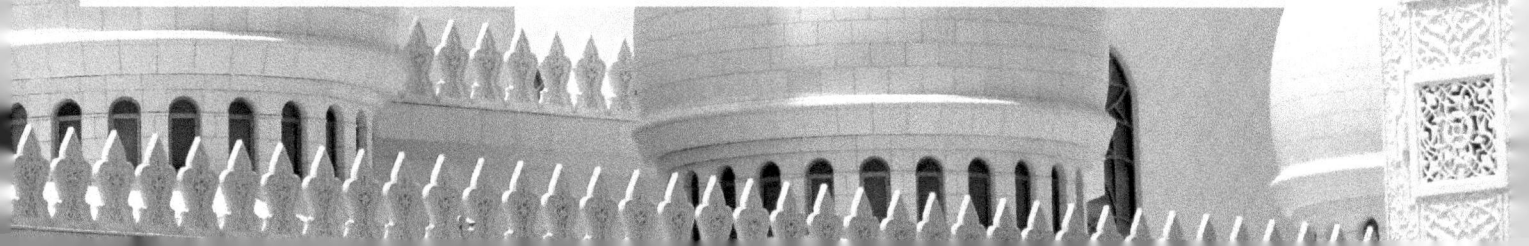

Introduction

This text is a follow-up to Volume 8 in the series that explains why manual and movement therapy practices are effective, and it also describes how they work at a cellular level. There are ways in which the critical information that is transmitted through the cellular matrix keeps our bodies in balance can be optimized and applied in daily life. That information will be offered here in this volume in the form of somatic movement sequences, sensory awareness prompts, and hands-on recommendations that can be used on yourself or with your clients/patients.

Along with the studies that showed how the cells performed optimally, Volume 8 also includes the many ways that optimum cellular interactions can be interfered with, resulting in all sorts of illnesses and premature aging. One fascinating article studied which tissues show signs of aging first – namely, the heart and cardiovascular system – which is supported by them being the number-one cause of death worldwide. The British Heart Foundation reported in 2023 that the global numbers of heart disease has doubled (to well over 600 million) since the 1990s. The American Heart Association estimated that over 19 million deaths in 2020 were attributed to heart disease. However, the heart doesn't exist in a vacuum.

Although we're speaking about which system or organ ages first, remember that all systems and organs are comprised of cells, and cells have varying rates and reasons for aging. Cells are interconnected, so changes in one system will impact the others. In general, there are four types of tissue: connective (supports, binds, and permeates other tissues), epithelial (covers and protects organs and vessels), muscle (striated and smooth), and nerve tissue (National Library of Medicine, Medline Plus, April,18, 2023). The rate of change can vary a great deal from one person to another. According to Medline Plus, a host of changes happen in the cells that affect the cell's ability to function properly or efficiently:

ONE SKY

Waste products accumulate as fatty/lipid molecules.

Connective tissue becomes stiffer, which inhibits the flow and exchange of information and substances, as well as repair or restoration activities.

Tissues then begin to lose or reflexively gain mass and may function more slowly.

Stressors like illness, life changes, medication, trauma, or environmental impacts take more of a toll and challenge the body's adaptability.

Cells begin changing their organization/shape, or increase in number (hyperplasia).

Cells begin to distort and form a benign or malignant mass.

Ye Ella Tan et al. finds that there can be a tremendous difference between the biological age of a system or organ and its chronological age. (Tian, et al., *"Heterogeneous aging across multiple organ systems and prediction of chronic disease and mortality,"* Nature Medicine; March, 2023){1} These researchers, using a large sample of over 143,000 participants from ages 39 to 82 found a significant relationship between organ age and brain age, with brain age having the strongest impact upon multiple organs. The cardiovascular system was shown to have the strongest impact on brain age, particularly the age of grey matter. That said, they also found that pulmonary age greatly affects cardiovascular age, and environmental factors are largely responsible for pulmonary age. Pulmonary age, according to this study, is the greatest predictor of mortality.

Chao Nie and his group used over 4000 subjects in their study and found that organs have multiple clocks and that people age differently, but that one main determining factor in aging and mortality is DNA methylation. (Nie, et al. Cell Reports, 2022){2} Their team narrowed down the markers to chromosome 6 as it relates to the immune function's impact on the cardiovascular system. They also noticed two specific pathways involved in DNA excision repair and a few signaling pathways (e.g. Notch, Hedgehog, VEGF, p53) that had become compromised, creating instability in the DNA that accelerate aging. Although signs of aging can be noticed in the early 20s, Nie and his team emphasize that it is a gradual systemwide cellular process that may appear or present as organ-specific.

An international team of researchers collaborated to publish an article in 2016 on the physiology of aging, focusing on metabolic processes as a predictor of longevity. They cite that the root cause of aging is the capacity of the cells to uptake oxygen and maintain balance between macromolecular damage and repair. (vanBeek, Kirkwood and Bassingthwaighte, *"Understanding the physiology of the ageing individual: computational modelling of changes in metabolism and endurance,"* Interface Focus, 2016){3} The team stated that, *"It is the efficacy of maintenance and repair processes which determine how long it takes for this eventual degradation to occur. ...If not repaired, the damage will accumulate and for instance lead to oxidation of DNA."*

This team asserts that metabolism and endurance are key factors in aging, which are cut in half by age 75. VanBeek also reports that, *"Metabolism provides not only energy by burning the carbohydrates and fats in our food, but also small, molecular building blocks, such as amino acids and fatty acids, which are used for synthesis of macromolecules such as proteins and lipids. Metabolism is therefore of enormous importance for muscle building and energy turnover."* Metabolism and its regulatory mechanisms also don't exist in a vacuum and they are vulnerable to our capacity to adapt to life's challenges.

Numerous preventative measures and modalities were discussed in Volume 8, so there's no need to repeat the results of those studies on what can protect against cell or DNA damage and improve homeostasis. We now know that movement in general and particularly conscious movement can create epigenetic changes by enhancing cellular communication and improving the structures that function in that capacity. The delivery of information, energy, and nourishment along with the export of waste are all improved through motion and in fact require movement to fulfill those duties accurately. Many feel that much of the delivery of information happens via the central nervous system and neurotrophic substances. Therefore, somatic pioneers and chiropractors, along with modern researchers, feel that the health of the CNS is key to the homeostasis of the other systems.

Remember that, as pointed out in Volume 8, our bodies function and communicate through an intricate matrix or cytoskeleton that is subject to and dependent on mechanical loads. These intricate structures are organized at smaller and smaller layers which are subject to the same forces that we perceive to be influencing our muscles, organs, connective tissue, fluids, and nerves. The ability for energetic production and transport or transmission happens only as permitted by the elasticity, permeability, slide and/or glide of these tissues. We can intentionally and consciously participate in the optimization of those qualities that are needed for accurate intercellular and intracellular communication, as will be illustrated throughout this book.

Initially, but only briefly, we'll address the main ways that the most important systems interact, as they've been shown to also be the first ones to show signs of wear, degeneration, and dysfunction. They are also formed first embryologically and have the most potential to reset and harmonize the rest of the body - the midline structures and their vital functions. It's not a coincidence that ancient traditions include these structures as a part of achieving and maintaining well-being because it's been known for thousands of years that they are the most restorative.

The movements and self-regulatory manual methods illustrated in this text will work from the basis of which systems have been shown to be the most influential upon the others, and which systems were developed first in the embryo. Although we will focus on the physical and neurophysiological aspects of the interdependent communication (mechanotransduction) processes at the molecular level that make these beneficial changes possible, the mental, emotional, and spiritual aspects of what makes us whole will always be implied. All of those levels, coincidentally, are processed by the heart.

These words are not designed to prove anything. The words express the awe and love I see in this beautiful living form – form that minute to minute wants to be balanced."

Dr. James Jealous

Chapter 1
The Heart of the Matter

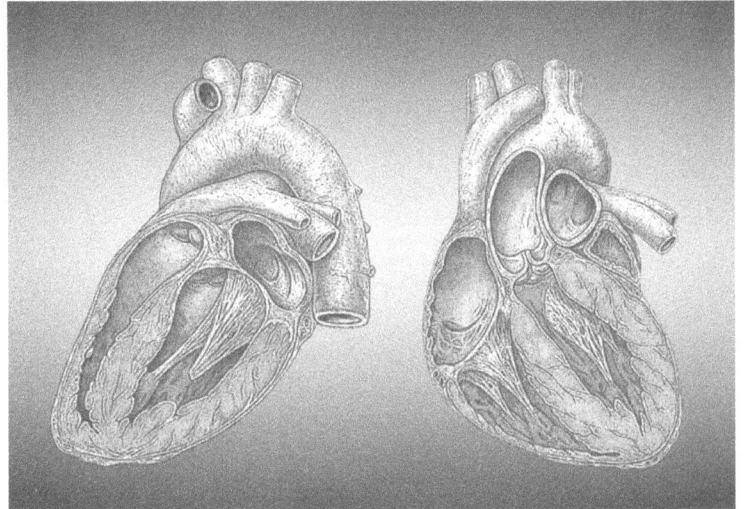

(Image courtesy of Helkenwaelder Hugo, helkenwaelder@aon.at, www.helkenwaelder.at, CC BY-SA 2.5 via Wikimedia Commons)

Sudden death in athletes

The heart plays such a significant role in what compromises health and well-being that it deserves to be a focus here. Later in the text we will address movement and self-regulatory practices to help protect it and prevent its decline. Gaining light in recent years are the athletes who suddenly drop dead on the football field or basketball court. It is the highest cause of sudden death in young athletes, with Black males being the most at risk. (Drs. Meagan Wasfy, Adolph Hutter, and Rory Weiner, "*Sudden Cardiac Death in Athletes*," Debakey-Journal XII (2) 2016){4] High school, college, and pro athletes alike are vulnerable to this scary situation, but pro basketball players are somehow the most at risk.

Congenital disorders or anomalies account for about 17% -25% of sudden cardiac death (SCD) cases, which may be slightly higher in other countries. According to this team of doctors, the increased risk group for collegiates as of 2023 is as follows:

Characteristic	Increased Risk Group	Decreased Risk Group
Gender	Males - 1 in 37,790	Females - 1 in 121,593
Race	Black - 1 in 21,491	White - 1 in 68,354
		Hispanic - 1 in 56,254
Sports	Men's basketball - 1 in 8,978	N/A
	Men's soccer - 1 in 23,689	
	Men's football - 1 in 35,951	

A recent study from Columbia University that examined over 500 hearts of players in the National Basketball Association found that these athletes had different hearts than the rest of the population (Fig.1.1). Considering the size of most players, this was to be expected. They also had larger aortas and larger left ventricles, which pump blood to the rest of the body. However, 25% of the players exhibited a thickening or hypertrophy of the left ventricle, which is a sign of decreasing heart function. ("Medical Research Studies NBA Players' Hearts," Black Health Matters.com, 2023)[5]

Some causes of sudden death

The sudden bursts of energy required in that sport can expose an underlying condition which may not have shown symptoms previously, reports sports medicine expert, Dr. Sara Gould. She goes on to recommend that the 14-point checklist from the American Heart Association be required for all players each year. (UABMedicine, "Basketball Players Suffer the Highest Rate of Sudden Cardiac Death," 2023){6} The Cleveland Clinic and others mention that high blood pressure can often lead to left ventricular hypertrophy (LVH) which is often found in SCD (Fig. 1.2). They also assert that the intense demands of certain sports can cause thickening of the walls due to the amount and rate of blood flow required. Certain changes are unavoidable, so regular monitoring is needed.

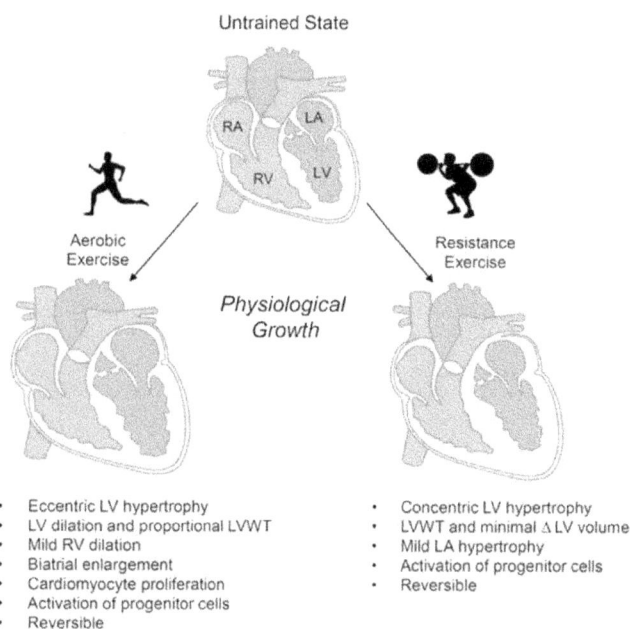

Untrained State

Aerobic Exercise

Resistance Exercise

Physiological Growth

- Eccentric LV hypertrophy
- LV dilation and proportional LVWT
- Mild RV dilation
- Biatrial enlargement
- Cardiomyocyte proliferation
- Activation of progenitor cells
- Reversible

- Concentric LV hypertrophy
- LVWT and minimal ∆ LV volume
- Mild LA hypertrophy
- Activation of progenitor cells
- Reversible

Fig. 1.1 – Changes in the heart based on physical exertion
Image courtesy of Steve Lipofsky at basketballphoto. com, CC BY-SA 3.0 via Wikimedia commons

Jennie Han and her team of researchers listed dehydration, an electrolyte imbalance, and acid/base disturbance as frequent results of intense exercise that can trigger an underlying arrhythmia and electrical dysfunction. (Han et.al, "Sudden Cardiac Death in Athletes: Facts and Fallacies," J Cardiovasc Dev Dis. 2023 Feb; 10(2): 68) [6} However, in athletes over age 35, many studies cite the more common cause as being artherosclerosis. It's theorized that women make up a smaller (58% vs. 83%) percentage of SCDs partially because they don't have the same tendency to push themselves to exhaustion or to demonstrate addictive tendencies in sports, they have less incidence of artherosclerosis, and because estrogen may be cardioprotective.

Autopsies were not conducted in all cases, some of the autopsies were not performed by a cardiologist, so the data on causes are educated hypotheses. Many who have been tracking SCD speculate that it happens every 5 days, or to one in 40,000 - 80,000 athletes. Some feel that the estimates are more accurate when looking at the military. An army cardiologist who published a study in 2004 found that 18 to 35 year-old male and female exercisers who expressed a risk were 1 in 15,000; about 20 times higher than what had previously been reported at that time. Dr. Robert Eckart felt those numbers were more accurate than sports estimates, which were largely relying on media reports for their information. Subsequent research in which autopsies were undergone revealed that, although a certain percentage of SCDs were caused by genetic defects or conditions, a large percentage had no anomalies in the heart and were unexplained.

Team physicians Jonathan Drezner and Kimberly Harmon have since set up a non-profit called the Nick of Time Foundation that screens up to 500 high school athletes per month and raises awareness about sudden cardiac death in young athletes. (Brian Mossop, *"Death on the Basketball Court,"* The New Yorker, 2014){7} In the general population, however, the numbers are much higher. Weight, diabetes, alcohol or tobacco use, and stress can be contributing factors when high-level sports are not concerned. In these cases, the numbers are as high as 950 deaths per day. (Semsarian, Ingles, and Wilde, *"Sudden cardiac death in the young: the molecular autopsy and a practical approach to surviving relatives,"* European Heart Journal (2105) 36, 1290-1296)[8]

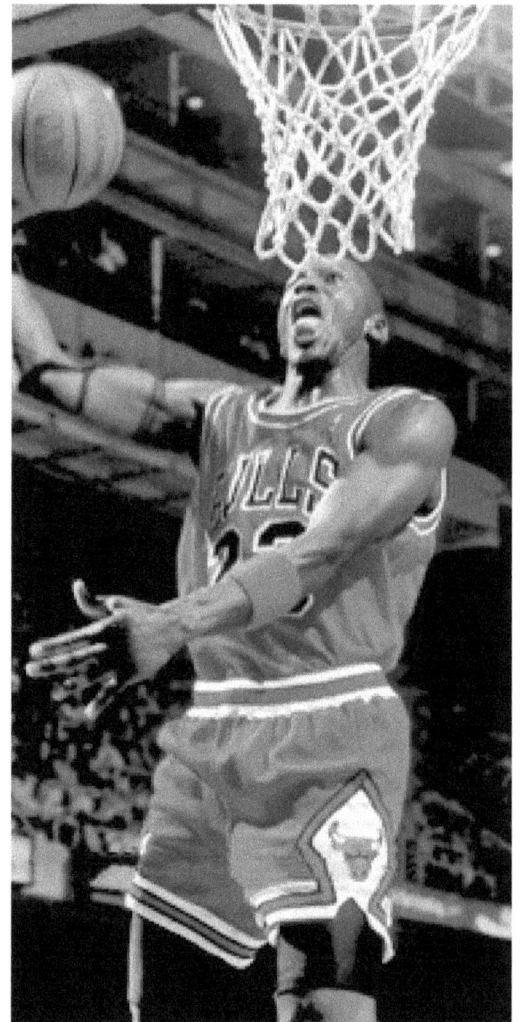

Courtesy of Kyle Fulghum and Bradford G. Hill, CC BY-SA 4.0 via Wikimedia Commons

Distinguishing breath disorders from heart issues

Doctors Emery (M.D.) and Milstein (PhD) stress the importance for sports cardiologists to distinguish breathing dysfunction from heart issues, which may appear symptomatically similar. Breathlessness, palpitations, dizziness, and chest pain could also be an indication of EIB (exercise-induced bronchoconstriction) or EILO, (exercise-induced laryngeal obstruction involving the vocal cords). These types of breathing pattern disorders (BPD) are apparently common in young athletes. (Michael Scott Emery, M.D. FACC; and Claudio Milstein, PhD, *"Dysfunctional Breathing in Athletes: A Brief Primer for the Sports Cardiologist,"* American College of Cardiology, May 11, 2022)[9] Studies have shown that **regular consumption of vitamin C reduces the incidence by nearly 50%,** and preserves the health of the lungs going forward, preventing decline. (*"Vitamin C: An Essential Nutrient for Good Lung and Respiratory Health,"* Respiratory Health, 19 March 2023)[10]

BPD symptoms most often develop during intense exercise and resolve rapidly on exercise cessation with the athlete commonly reporting difficulty breathing in and/or an inability to get a complete breath in.

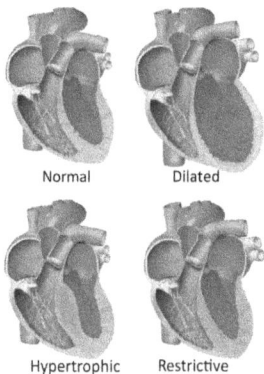

Normal   Dilated

Hypertrophic   Restrictive

Fig. 1.2 – *Normal vs. damaged heart 1*

Each of these conditions involves dysfunctional inhalation muscles, that result in coughing, wheezing, tightness in the throat or chest, or in difficulty 'catching one's breath'. EILO is more common in females, is brought on by exercise, and doesn't respond to inhalers. It may become coupled with EIB, or with anxiety and hyperventilation and can occur as frequently as in one-third of athletes. These authors report hypertonicity in the neck along with thoraco-abdominal asynchrony, often accompanied by a pattern of chest breathing. Emery and Milstein recommend a cardiopulmonary exercise test in order to distinguish breath disorders from those related to heart failure.

Common congenital heart disorders

The list of congenital heart conditions that may be contributing to sudden death is fairly long. It is the most common area in which congenital defects arise. Among them are:

- ➲ Hypertrophic cardiomyopathy
- ➲ Dilated and constrictive cardiomyopathies
- ➲ Arrhythmic right ventricular cardiomyopathy
- ➲ Long QT syndrome
- ➲ Short QT syndrome
- ➲ Brugada syndrome (electrical)

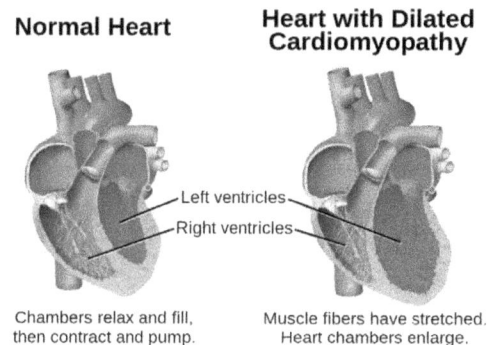

Normal Heart   **Heart with Dilated Cardiomyopathy**

Left ventricles
Right ventricles

Chambers relax and fill, then contract and pump.

Muscle fibers have stretched. Heart chambers enlarge.

Fig. 1.3 – *Normal vs. damaged heart 2*
Fig. 1.2 - Image courtesy of Blausen.com staff (2014). "Medical gallery of Blausen Medical 2014." WikiJournal of Medicine 1(2)DOI:10. 15347/w/m/2014 010. ISSN 2002-4438, CC BY-SA 3.0 via Wikimedia Commons; and Fig. 1.3 - Courtesy of Npathcett, CC BY-SA 4.0, via Wikimedia Commons

➲ Left ventricular non-compaction

➲ Idiopathic ventricular fibrillation

➲ Marfan syndrome (connective tissue disorder)

➲ Vascular Ehlers-Danlos syndrome (connective tissue disorder)

➲ Loeys-Dietz Syndrome (connective tissue disorder)

➲ Catecholaminergic polymorphic ventricular tachycardia

➲ Septal defects

The arrhythmogenic disorders don't create a change in the appearance of the heart, which makes it more difficult to ascertain the cause of death in an autopsy. Christopher Semsarian et al. speculated that these 'unknown causes' make up about 30% of sudden death cases. These researchers hypothesize that many motorcycle accidents and cases of drowning involving good swimmers could have been preceded by a ventricular arrhythmia in patients with a family history of such disorders. Volume 8 went into detail about the period between day 18 and 50 of a pregnancy when the heart of the fetus is developing. It is critical to the health of the person's heart throughout life.

Besides medications the mother may be taking, dietary fat, electrolyte imbalance, blood sugar, and stress levels, the alcohol consumption and smoking by the father greatly increased the risk of congenital heart disease in the infant, especially electrical issues. This is a particularly tricky time for all concerned, because it often isn't clear that there is a pregnancy before 6 or 8 weeks, when much of this process has already been underway. Preventative measures are always best, but there have been several natural means of helping to mitigate heart conditions that have achieved success.

Preventative and protective measures for the heart

In 2016, Yvette Brazier quoted a finding reported in the Journal of the American Heart Association stating that both **T'ai Chi** (Fig. 1.4) **and Chi Kung** can "boost the well-being of people with cardiovascular disease, high blood pressure, or stroke." (Yvette Brazier, *"Chinese exercise is good for the heart,"* Medical News Today, March 10, 2016) [11] Lauren Bedosky also found in her review of studies on Chi Kung that the gentle repetitive movements can help circulation as well as stimulate a parasympathetic response that settles the nervous system, reduces stress and lowers blood pressure. (Lauren Bedosky, *"6 Potential Health Benefits of Qigong – A TCM Mind-Body Practice,"* Everyday Health, June 15, 2022)[12]

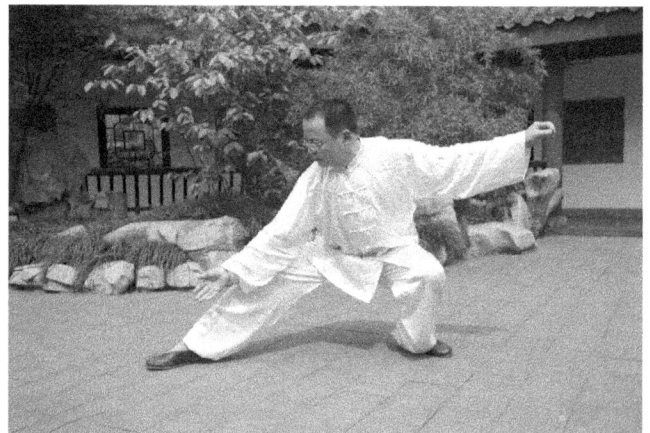

Fig.1.4 - *T'ai Chi Movement*
Courtesy of Sarvodaya Shramadana from Colombo,

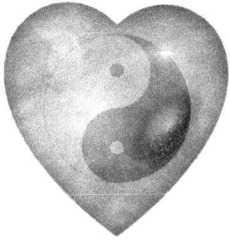

Another article quoted the results of several studies on this ancient Asian art, saying, "From high blood pressure to cardiac rehabilitation, this Ancient Chinese practice of Qi Gong has been known to strengthen and revitalize the heart." (Michelle Fletcher, B.A., *"Strengthen the Heart with Qi Gong,"* Pacific College of Health and Science, 2023)[13] She goes on to say that the art itself combines isometrics, isotonics, breathing exercises, aerobic conditioning, relaxation, an inward focus, balance, and meditation. However, I know a tai chi instructor who practices meditation and still needed triple bypass surgery. When I asked him what happened to cause it, he admitted that he often ate at McDonalds, so diet is a big factor in all of this. The grace for him in this was that he had a heart attack during a stress test in the cardiologist's office.

Meditation and mindfulness have been studied for many years and both have proven to have a positive effect on the brain and the heart. **Meditation** can also have a positive effect on heart rate variability (HRV). HRV reflects how quickly your heart can make little adjustments in between each heartbeat. It's been shown that low HRV provides a 32% to 45% increased risk of heart attack or stroke among those who do not have cardiovascular disease. Just 5 minutes/day of meditation for 10 days increases heart rate variability.

Moving meditations like Tai Chi, Chi Kung, **Feldenkrais, Hanna Somatics**, or **Yoga** can be as beneficial as meditating without motion. (Harvard Health Medical School, *"Mindfulness can improve heart health,"* Feb. 1, 2018) [14] Nine studies involving over 500 participants revealed that Tai Chi and Chi Kung exercise practiced over a few months were able to reduce both diastolic and systolic blood pressure values along with increasing blood levels of nitric oxide. (Liu, et al, Evid. Based Complement Alternat Med 2020; 2020 Jul 30)[15]

Nitric oxide (NO) relaxes blood vessel walls and is released from the walls (endothelium) themselves during exercise. Enhanced levels of NO increase nutrient absorption, improve circulation and microcirculation, and reduce the risk of cardiovascular disease. (Tahereh Arefirad, et al., *"Effect of exercise training on nitric oxide and nitrate/nitrite (NOx) production: A systematic review and meta-analysis,"* Frontiers in Physiology, 04 October 2022)[16] These researchers, after narrowing down thousands of articles to a dozen that matched their criteria, found an increased level of NO production regardless of the type (aerobic or anaerobic), duration, or intensity of the workout. Blood lipids, blood sugar, and blood pressure all benefit from exercise.

Tai Chi, yoga, and chi kung are uniquely suited to provide extra benefits of calming the nervous system through mindfulness and increasing balance and coordination while building strength. It is likely that incorporating slowed-down movement practices will also increase focus, alignment, and execution for professional athletes, offering greater protection for their overall health. It's a fact that legendary coach, Phil Jackson, integrated some spiritual aspects into the training of his teams, including the one with MVP Kobe Bryant. (Arjun Julka, The Sports Rush, May 14, 2022)[16]

More studies are needed to measure how much mindful movement can reduce the incidence of SCD. Tai Chi has been shown to be cardio-protective. A study of 120 adults over 50 years of age over a 5-year period showed that the group practicing tai chi had significantly lower blood pressure, (Fig.1.5) were more than half as likely to develop cardiac disease, and also had significantly higher lung function than the control group. (Lei Sun, MD, et al, "Tai Chi can prevent cardiovascular disease and improve cardiopulmonary function of adults with obesity aged 50 years and older," Medicine, 2019 Oct; 98(42))[17]

Stress and the heart

Dr. Michelle Dossett, a physician and researcher at the Benson-Henry Institute compiled data from 4000 medical records where their doctors recommended yoga, tai chi, and meditation for stress relief over an 8-year period. Compared to 13,000 patients whose doctors didn't make those recommendations, the **mindful exercise** group were 43% less likely to visit the hospital, need medical tests or emergency room care than the group who didn't use those means of movement. According to these researchers, stress-related issues account for between 75% and 90% of all doctor visits. (Carolyn Gregoire, "*Yoga and Meditation Shown to Drastically Reduce Hospital Visits,*" Science, October 28, 2016)[18]

Massage and manual therapy can also significantly reduce stress and settle the nervous system, help balance tissue fields, fluid systems and joints, as well as open the flow of energetic systems that feed all of the above. A review of 78 articles on the subject involving animals, reported that joint mobilization induced "changes in nociceptive (pain) and inflammatory profiles, gene expression, receptor activation, neurotransmitter release, and enzymatic activity."

They found that **spinal manipulation** produced "*changes in muscle spindle response, nocifensive reflex response (reaction to discomfort) and neuronal activity, electromyography (nerve to muscle response), and immunologic responses.*" Simulated (in vitro) **massage** produced physiological changes involving autonomic, circulatory, lymphatic, visceral, and immunologic functions, along with gene expression, neuroanatomical and cellular responses. (Lima, Martins, and Reed, "*Physiological Responses Induced by Manual Therapy in Animal Models: a Scoping Review,*" Frontiers in Neuroscience, 08 May 2020){19} Certain types of massage may be counter-indicated for those with Afib, with pacemakers, or for those who are on blood thinners.

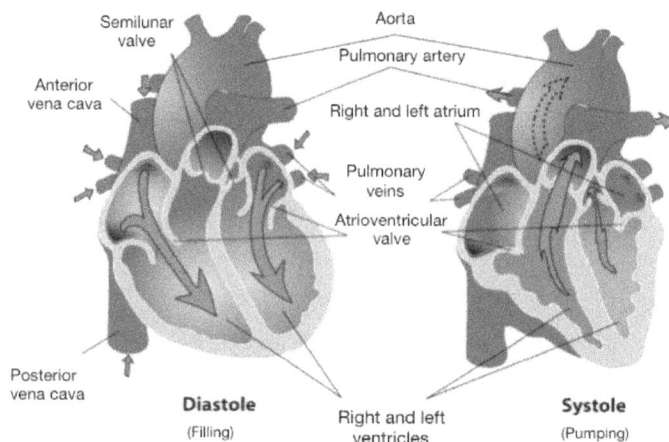

Fig. 1.5 – *Both diastolic and systolic readings decreased significantly after tai chi and qigong exercises. (Courtesy of LadyofHats, Public domain via Wikimedia Commons)*

*"Cardiac remodeling comprises changes in heart structure such as alterations in cardiac wall thickness, chamber size, cell dimension, cell number, and extracellular matrix volume. These structural changes can influence heart function. **Hawthorn** markedly reduced LV chamber volumes (VOL) after aortic constriction (AC) and augmented relative wall thickness and attenuated the AC-induced decrease in velocity of circumferential shortening (Vcfc) showing anti left ventricular remodeling and antimyocardial dysfunction in early pressure overload-induced cardiac hypertrophy."* (Hudson, 2014)[20]

Herbal remedies for the heart

A few herbs have been shown over time to be helpful and protective for heart issues. **Hawthorn** (Crataegus monogyna) berries, flowers, and leaves are known for their ability to function like a tonic for the heart, possibly due to the high content of flavonoids, particularly proanthocyanidin. Numerous studies have shown that hawthorn can dilate coronary artery blood vessels, somewhat decrease blood pressure, and slightly increase the heart's muscle contractions, facilitating better tolerance for exercise. It has also been shown to significantly improve angina and achieve better outcomes for those with compromised left ventricular ejection fraction. (Tori Hudson, ND, *"Hibiscus, Hawthorne, and the Heart,"* Natural Medicine Journal, March 22, 2014)[20]

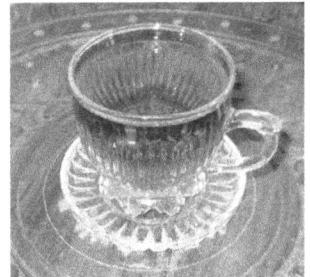

Fig. 1.6 – *Hibiscus tea Courtesy of MRG90 CC BY-SA via Wikimedia Commons*

Hudson also reviewed numerous studies regarding the efficacy of **hibiscus tea** (Hibiscus sabdariffa), which also contains polyphenols and anthocyanins, including quercetin and protocatechuic acid - a powerful antioxidant, anti-inflammatory, and anti-hyperglycemic agent. Throughout the various studies, with varying dosages being used by hundreds of participants, hibiscus consistently lowered systolic blood pressure levels, raised HDL cholesterol, lowered blood sugar, and often lowered LDL and total cholesterol levels. Each of these functions can potentially be protective for the heart. There are dozens of species of hibiscus, and it might be worth investigating which are the most beneficial for the heart.

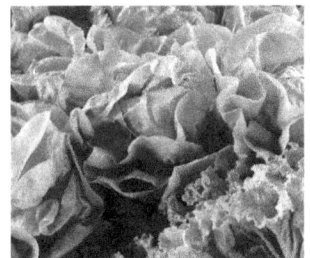

Fig. 1.75 – *Leafy greens Courtesy of Mark Stebnicki and Pexels*

There are well over 100 species of hawthorn, and one group of researchers chose Crataegus **oxyacantha** for their study. The list of properties it has shown to possess include: inotropic (alters the force or energy of muscular contractions) effect, anti-inflammatory effect, anticardiac remodeling effect, antiplatelet aggregation effect, vasodilating effect, endothelial protective effect, reduction of smooth muscle cell migration and proliferation, protective effect against ischemia/reperfusion injury, antiarrhythmic effect, lipid-lowering effect, and decreased arterial blood pressure effect along with being an antioxidant. These potential benefits have placed it under scrutiny for its use in heart failure, hypertension, and high cholesterol.

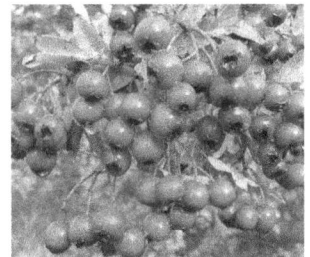

Fig. 1.7 Hawthorne berries
Courtesy of Andrew Smith

Doctors Wang, Xiong, and Feng, from the Department of Cardiology at the Guang'anmen Hospital in Beijing report that the oxyacantha variety is most popular for its cardio-protective effects. Dysfunctional cardiac remodeling following a heart attack or progressive disease can become a significant factor in fatalities, and hawthorn may be helpful in this category. In any research cited, the results were based on a specific dose over a period of time.

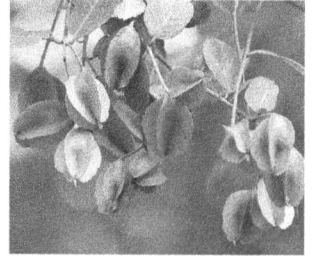

Fig. 1.80 – *Arjuna Courtesy of J.M. Garg, CC BY-SA 3.0 Via Wikimedia Commons*

These researchers also cited studies of over 2600 patients (1300 with hawthorn, 1300 with a placebo) when a **standardized hawthorn extract** was tested as an adjunct to other heart medications. The group using hawthorn reduced sudden cardiac death by over 39%. Wang et al. in particular recommended hawthorn oxyacantha for the early stages of heart failure and support more rigorous studies for its use in high blood pressure and high cholesterol. It has been used in China for many health conditions for many generations. (Jie Wang, Xingjjang Xiong, Bo Feng, *"Effect of Crataegus in Cardiovascular Disease Prevention: an Evidence-Based Study,"* Evidence Based Complementary and Alternative Medicine, November, 2013)[21]

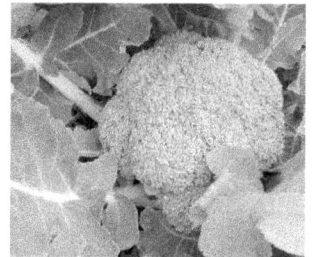

Fig. 1.85 – *Broccoli Courtesy of Creative Commons- Share Alike 3.0 Unported*

Gallic acid is a common polyphenol found in most parts of many types of plants, including berries, cocoa, yams, green leafy vegetables, broccoli, spices, certain grains, nuts, and citrus. It is a powerful antioxidant that is neuroprotective and cardioprotective. It also has a protective role in plants, defending them against parasites, pathogens, and radiation. (Jin Dai and Russell J. Mumper, *"Plant Phenolics: Extraction, analysis and Their Antioxidant and Anticancer Properties,"* Molecules, 2010 Oct; 15(10) 7313-7352)[22]

In 2018, Lin Jin and a team of researchers discovered that, "Gallic acid reduces cardiac hypertrophy, dysfunction, and fibrosis induced by transverse aortic constriction (TAC) stimuli in vivo and transforming growth factor ß1 (TGF-ß1) in vitro. The study was performed on mice, which have hearts that are remarkably similar to human hearts and have DNA that is 97.5% the same. In vivo gallic acid decreases left ventricular end-diastolic and end-systolic diameter, and recovers the reduced fractional shortening in TAC." (Lin Jin, et al., *"Gallic acid improves cardiac dysfunction and fibrosis in pressure overload-induced heart failure,"* Scientific Reports, 18 June 2018)[23]

They also reported that gallic acid, in their tests, performed better than a few drugs currently on the market to treat hypertrophy and fibrosis that accompany hypertension and heart failure. **Arjuna Terminalia** (Fig. 1.8), an Ancient Ayurvedic remedy contains both gallic and ellagic acids and has traditionally been used as a heart tonic. It has been known to lower blood pressure, dilate blood vessels, improve coronary artery blood flow, strengthen the heart muscle, and help prevent ischemic damage. (Somya Binu, MSc., *"Arjuna: This Herbal Hero Protects Your Heart Health,"* netmeds.com, September 13. 2021)[24] It is rich in CoQ10, which supports heart function, and can also lower LDL cholesterol levels.

(Dr. Vikram Chauhan, "*Arjuna – Best Herb for Heart Care*," Planet Ayurveda, August 8, 2023){25} Regarding any type of herbal remedy, results will be dependent upon the dose applied over time, which may vary for each individual.

The adult human heart may have limited abilities to regenerate itself, particularly after an injury, which makes it more important to be proactive in caring for it. Cardiac cells do regenerate somewhat after birth, but only at the rate of 1% per year up to age 75, and even less after that. (Wade, 2009, Mason, 2014) Millions of heart cells perish during a heart attack, so it's very difficult to replace them all, which makes the herbal protection that reduces scarring even more important to consider.

Oral health and heart disease

An article in the Penn Heart and Vascular blog in May 2022 stated that, "*Researchers suspect that bacteria present in gum disease can travel throughout the body, triggering inflammation in the heart's vessels and (trigger) infection in heart valves.*" It is estimated that almost half of Americans over age 30 have some form of gum disease. Researchers in the UK, after reviewing several studies following over 2000 participants that spanned several years, found that both British and American citizens over middle age with **dry mouth, tooth loss, or periodontal disease** had an increase in all-cause mortality as well as cardiovascular and lung issues. (Eftychia Kotronia, et al., "*Oral health and all-cause cardiovascular disease, and respiratory mortality in older people in the UK and USA*," Scientific Reports, 2021)[26]

A study in the Journal of Dental Research published in 2016 reports that people with **untreated tooth infections** have nearly three times the risk of developing heart disease. Red, painful, swollen, bleeding gums are sure signs of inflammation that should stimulate a visit to the dentist. On the other hand, a 2018 study of over a million people who'd experienced heart disease, the correlation disappeared after smoking was eliminated from the criteria. The correlation shifted, but not the connection. There have been sufficient studies to link periodontal disease to rheumatoid arthritis and even pancreatic cancer, as pertains to the porphyromonas gingivalis bacteria, so those that connect it to heart disease aren't all wrong, but it may not stand alone as a cause. (Robert H. Shmerling, MD, "*Gum disease and the connection to heart disease*," Harvard Health Publishing, April 22, 2021){27}

The **visceral and vascular aspects** of the embryo are both derived from the **splanchnic layer** of the lateral plate mesoderm. (Fig.1.9) They are born out of the same cells and by nature are interrelated, as are the foregut and the lungs. This may be why, in Traditional Chinese Medicine, the lung and large intestine meridians are paired, as are the heart and small intestine. Structurally, the cells of the gut tube (the foregut) and the developing heart are just millimeters away from one another (Fig.1.10). That said, certain bacteria in the gut can also affect the adult heart as well as the brain. We now know that there are tens of thousands of neurons in the heart, that there is an enteric nervous system, and that the vagus nerve directly influences all internal organs. As emphasized in Volume 8, the ectoderm (brain, skin, and central nervous system layers) interpenetrates the endoderm and mesoderm.

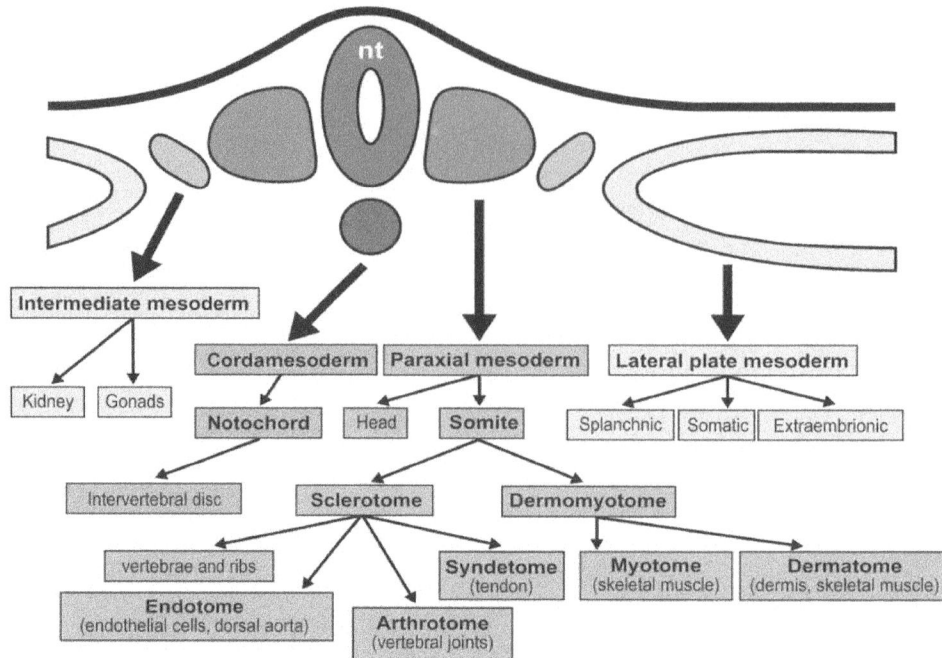

Fig. 1.9 - - Initial formation of the mesodermal layers in the embryo's first weeks, out of which the internal organs, skeleton, connective tissue, and limbs are formed. (nt = neural tube)
Image courtesy of Creative Commons Attribution 4.0 International

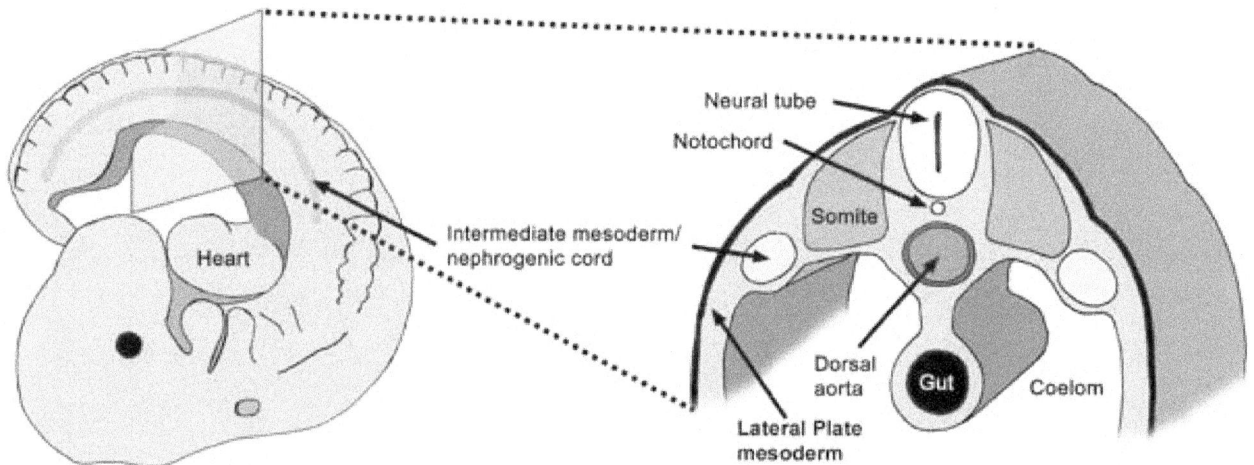

Fig. 1.10 – *Illustrating the unfolding of the lateral plate mesoderm derivatives in the embryo, whereby the neural tube, heart tubes (dorsal aorta), and gut tube are separated only by millimeters as countless complex transcriptions processes occur along numerous signaling pathways to express their fate. (Axel H. Newton, et. al, 2022; Bruce M. Carlson MD, PhD, 2014; Kristen L. Farraj and Roman Zeltser, 2023)*
Image Courtesy of Davidson, A.J. Mouse kidney development (January 15, 2009) StemBook, ed. The Stem Cell Research Community, StemBook, doi/10.3824/stembook.org, CC BY 3.0, via Wikimedia Commons

These organs are being formed simultaneously with their epithelial tissues and cavities, creating a continuous mechanical interplay of communication between them. (Lu Han, et al., *"Single cell transcriptomics identifies a signaling network coordinating endoderm and mesoderm diversification during foregut organogenesis,"* Nature Communications, 2020)[28] It is possible that the internal organs play a much wider role than we realize in our comfort level day-to-day even in the absence of disease conditions. Jean-Pierre Barral estimates that up to 80% of muscular discomfort is due to internal organ issues.

Blood and lymphatic vessels as well as nerves are all considered to be connective tissue, not just ligaments and tendons or fascia. Those initial formative weeks describe functional interactions better than the way modern medicine divides systems into specialties, which can be misleading. These interrelationships also have emotional implications which is being acknowledged more often by some parts of the medical community. Bruno Bordini as his co-authors on the subject stated that:

> *The fascial unity influences not only movement but also emotions. Dysfunction of the fascial system that is perpetuated in everyday movements can cause an emotional alteration of the person. This emotional alteration could be originating from constant myofascial nonphysiological afferents, which would bring the emotional state and myofascial pathology to the same level… and the presence of myofascial alterations leads to postural alterations. (Bordoni, et al., National Library of Medicine, July 17, 2023)[29]*

Regeneration and the heart

It's crucial for health to protect the heart due to its limited powers of rejuvenation. One theory for this limited regeneration of the heart, is that once it needs to adapt to its outer environment (after birth), it reduces the number of nuclear pores—or pathways into the nucleus of the cell—along with the signalling protein, MAPK, in order to protect itself (Fig.1.11). With this reduction in signalling pathways, when high blood pressure happens, the heart is more protected from structural changes. This change, however, also limits the signals required for regeneration. (Han, et al., *"Changes in nuclear pore numbers control nuclear import and stress response of mouse hearts,"* Developmental Cell, Vol. 67, Issue 20, P2397-2411, October 24, 2022)[30]

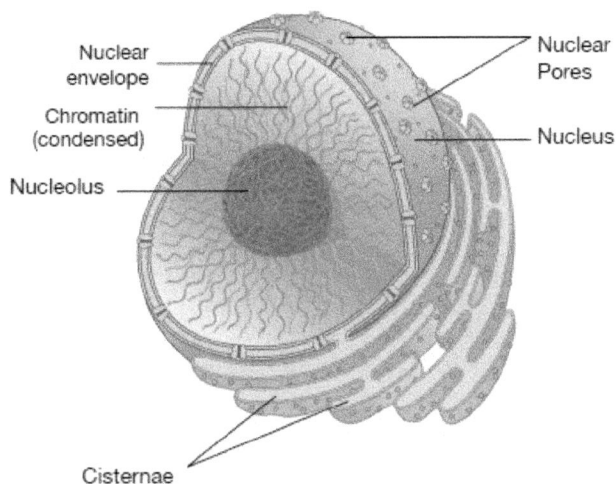

Fig. 1.11 – *Illustration of nuclear pores that are reduced by 63% within days of childbirth.*
Courtesy of OpenStax CC BY 4.0 via Wikimedia Commons

A novel and recent interpretation of why there is minimal cardiomyocyte cell division after 7 days of age, according to a large team of researchers at the University of Texas Southwestern Medical Center, is that the **fetal heart uses glucose** (anaerobic glycolysis) in utero, and must switch post-natal to using oxygen-dependent mitochondrial oxidative phosphorylation for the fatty acids in breast milk. Along with reduced protection from structural changes, the heart also has less protection from free radicals that damage mitochondria. (Alisson C. Cardoso, et al., *"Mitochondrial substrate utilization regulates cardiomyocyte cell-cycle progression,"* Nature Metabolism, Vol. 2 February 2020, 167-178)[31] These researchers determined using detailed analyses that **although fatty acids are the best method of energy production, they compromise the life span of the heart**.

The proliferation window in young mouse hearts was prolonged by offering a low-fat diet, and the reduced fatty acid intake was compensated for by increased production in the liver. It's clear that dietary fat and/or obesity puts the fetus at risk for congenital heart issues, and adult obesity is a factor in adult heart failure, but eliminating fats from the diet isn't productive. Rather, it's the type of fats (discussed in Volume 8) that make the difference. There are other dietary options to protect the heart. Ana Catarina Silva and her team of researchers reported that following a cardiac insult or injury resulting in cardiomyocyte death, there is a response by the extracellular matrix (ECM) that triggers a three-phase response: inflammation, proliferation, and maturation.

During the inflammatory phase, several cell types are activated for the repair process and to remove dead or damaged cells, which signal the proliferation phase to begin. Matricellular proteins enrich the ECM and coordinate the phenotype and deposit of various growth factors and structural proteins. Matricellular proteins are meant to protect the integrity of the walls of the heart, but something happens during this stage that isn't clearly understood as yet. The increase in collagen production without sufficient enzyme presence to establish a balance in the matrix enables rigid **scar tissue** to form that **restricts elasticity and electrical signalling**, potentially leading to heart failure. (Ana Catarina Silva, et al., *"Bearing My Heart: The Role of Extracellular Matrix on Cardiac Development, Homeostasis, and Injury Response,"* Frontiers in Cell and Developmental Biology, 12 January 2021)[32]

It's possible that herbal intervention could help correct these signalling snafus and establish a more balanced result. A few other herbs and spices that may help the heart remain healthy include garlic, fennel, cinnamon, magnolia bark, cardamom, ginger, resveratrol, green tea, ginseng, olive leaf, and turmeric. (Mohiuddin, 2019; Gupta, 2015) Their main mechanisms of action involve lowering blood pressure, lowering blood sugar and cholesterol levels, providing protection against inflammation and oxidation, reducing inappropriate clotting risks, and protecting vessel walls. Managing diet, exercise, and stress levels are the most popular narratives delivered to the public on this subject, but being more diligent and self-aware about which way to exercise and how to mitigate stress and trauma may be more beneficial than general recommendations. In any case, it's best to consult with an expert and listen to your body.

Cardioplasticity

Even though the heart may not be able to regenerate cardiomyocytes in great numbers or at significant speeds, it is adaptive. It can shift its size, energy-dependent remodeling of the major components of the myocyte, angiogenic alterations in blood supply, and more. (Gondalia, et. al, *"Cardiac Plasticity in Health and Disease,"* Translational Cardiology, January, 2012)[33]

> *A new paradigm, considering cardiomyocytes as highly plastic cells that rapidly respond to changes in their environment to enhance survival is emerging. Cardiomyocytes are remarkably resilient to damage, are able to survive several decades, often the whole life, despite relentless and constantly varying function." Watson, Perbellini, and Terracciano, "Cardiac t-tubules: where structural plasticity meets functional adaptation", Cardiovascular Research (2016) 112, 423-425[34]*

The heart contains a variety of types of cells, varying at times by location. According to Litviňuková in her original article on the subject, *Atrial tissues contain 30.1% cardiomyocytes, 24.3% fibroblasts, 17.1% mural cells (pericytes and vascular smooth muscle cells), 12.2% endothelial cells and 10.4% immune cells (myeloid and lymphoid). By contrast, ventricular tissues contain 19.2% cardiomyocytes, 21.2% mural cells, 15.5% fibroblasts, 7.8% endothelial cells, and 5.3% immune cells.* (Gregory Lim, *Complexity and plasticity of cardiac cellular composition,* Cell Biology, Nature Reviews/Cardiology, Volume 17, December 2020)[35]

These researchers also noted that the atrial and ventricular cardiomyocytes had different transcription signatures and different electrophysiological, contractile, and secretory properties. There were also numerous different categories or types of fibroblasts, immune cell and vascular endothelial cell populations. Additionally, they are not the same among men and women, in that some of the cellular distributions are regulated by endocrine factors. Lim cautions that much of the biomedical research trials are based on the phenotypes found in males, which are significantly different than those in females.

Pitoulis and Terraciano mention examples of short-term adaptive functioning of the heart in response to biochemical changes. For example, the flight/flight/freeze responses in the face of danger, chronic remodeling/plasticity in athletes like long-term rowers and skiers, and even pregnancy, which can alter the ventricular mass due to volume loads that revert after childbirth. They describe that cardiac plasticity is "a complex and multifactorial process." Its response involves metabolic, mechanical, electrical, and structural alterations and is known as cardiac plasticity. (*Fotius G. Pitoulis and Cesare M. Terracciano, "Heart Plasticity in Response to Pressure and Volume-Overload. A Review of Findings in Compensated and Decompensated Phenotypes,"* Frontiers in Physiology, 13 February 2020)[36] They go on to report that,

> *A decrease in systolic blood pressure decreases systolic load and is met with hormonal release, including angiotensin II and catecholamines. These not only modulate the function of the heart, but that of the vasculature as well, which in turn has mechanical consequences on the operation of the heart. Complex feedback loops are established in this manner, fine tuning the acute functional outputs of the heart while simultaneously driving remodeling. The adult human heart has an exceptional ability to alter its phenotype to adapt to changes in environmental demand.*

Whichever system we will speak about, it will be shown to be sensitive and responsive at the cellular level, literally to every move and decision we make. What we do in our daily lives, including how we use our bodies, drives those responses. Everyone has a different history that forms their heart, as well as being different in the experiences that shape it throughout life. Those same experiences shape posture, tension, and injury patterns. Self-sensing and self-regulation will always support self-knowledge. It's been shown over millennia that gentle, conscious movement holds countless benefits, and this text will take those benefits down into the universe of the sensorium—the body's internet system.

Being present in your sensorium—where sensory information is perceived, transmitted, and responded to—is where the magic happens. It is where your body wakes up to reveal the interconnections that are responsible for how and what you feel. While it can go into yogic proportions of superhuman feats, we don't need to take it that far to build a healthy dialogue with our sensory apparatus in a way that exponentially improves our quality of life. Just remember to consider that although these innermost layers are being activated all the time, just like the larger, more easily accessible systems, these deeper ones can also be awakened and more fully participate when gentler, very slow, conscious movements are done.

Within that is the fact that everything at every level in our body responds to the communication that happens through movement. The chest and abdominal cavities are packed with organs, fat, tissues, fluids, nerves, and blood vessels that are continuously interacting with one another. The mere proximity makes it a key area to consider regarding heart health and the pressures that can be exerted through neighboring structures. Very few researchers focus on the biomechanical and fascial relationships among the organs, but there is a well- known, inextricable relationship between the heart and the lungs (Fig. 1.12), and an implied one between the heart, lungs, and diaphragm.

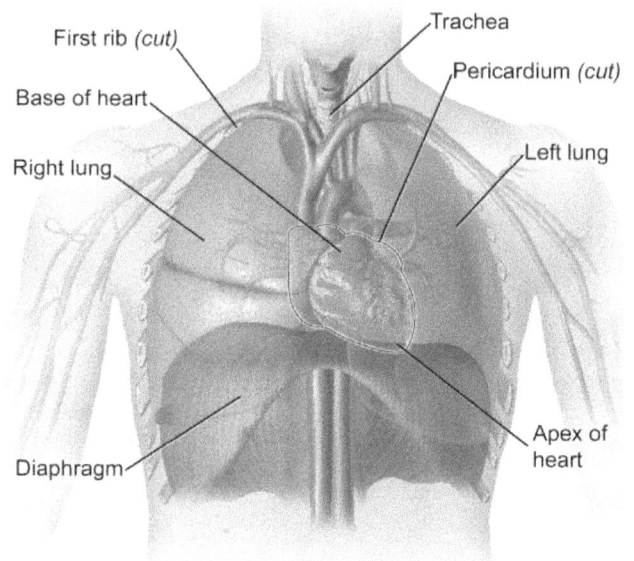

Location of Heart in Thoracic Cavity

Fig. 1.12: *Heart and lungs*
Blausen.com staff (2014). "Medical gallery of Blausen Medical 2014." WikiJournal of Medicine 1(2)DOI:10. 15347/w/m/2014 010. ISSN 2002-4436, CC BY-SA 3.0 via Wikimedia Commons

Interactions of the heart, muscles of respiration, and lungs

Troy James Cross et al. stated that, *The heart and lungs are intimately linked. These two organs interact with each other via hemodynamic (shared blood flow), mechanical, and neurohumoral (sympathetic activation including vasoconstrictive, vasodilation and cytokine factors) pathways. Thus, by virtue of these interrelationships, the presence of chronic disease or maladaptive changes in one organ system can markedly influence the health and function of the other.* (Troy James Cross, Chui-Ho Kim, Bruce D.

Johnson, and Sophie Lalande, *The interactions between respiratory and cardiovascular systems in systolic heart failure*, Journal of Applied Physiology, 128: 214-224, 2020)[37]

According to these researchers, heart failure patients breathe too much during exercise and tend to hyperventilate, loading the muscles of inspiration. A review of 13 studies on diaphragmatic deep breathing using 6 to10 breaths per minute for 10 minutes per day was effective in reducing hypertension, reducing sympathetic activity and increasing baroreflex sensitivity. (Katherine Ka-Yin Yau and Alice Yuen Loke, *Effects of diaphragmatic deep breathing exercises for prehypertensive or hypertensive adults: A literature review*, Complement. Ther. Clin. Pract., 2021 May) [38]

The Cleveland Clinic also reports that **chest breathing** is part of the problem in heart failure and lists the same benefits of diaphragmatic breathing as Yau and Loke in that it:

1. Facilitates relaxation
2. Improves muscle function during exercise preventing strain
3. Increases the level of oxygen in the blood
4. Facilitates the body releasing gas waste from the body
5. Reduces blood pressure
6. Reduces heart rate
7. Reduces stress and anxiety
8. May improve asthma and COPD

There are several muscles involved in respiration. The main muscles of inspiration, which elevate the rib cage and sternum, are the diaphragm and external intercostals. The accessory muscles also involved during inhalation are the sternocleidomastoid, scalenes, pectoralis major and minor, inferior fibers of the serratus anterior and latissimus dorsi, along with the serratus posterior superior and iliocostalis cervicus. (Rachel Lowe, *"Muscles of Respiration,"* Physiopedia, 2023)[39] Although expiration is mostly passive owing to the elastic recoil of the lungs, forceful expiration is accomplished by the internal intercostals, intercostalis intimi, subcostals, and the abdominal muscles (Fig. 1.14).

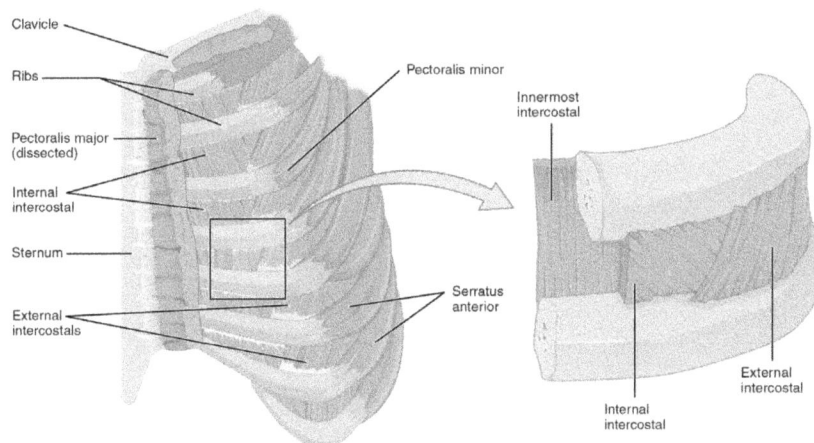

Fig. 1.13 – *Cross-section of the rib cage*

ONE SKY

Lesser known muscles are the transversus thoracis (deep anterior chest wall muscles), and levatores costarum (deep posterior chest wall muscles), that also help rotate and side bend the thoracic spine. These muscles can be influenced by posture, our daily activities, our mental/emotional status, and by our breathing patterns. It's helpful for whatever movement sequence you'd be using to take the several layers of intercostal muscles into consideration (Fig. 1.13), along with the intrinsic nerve and blood supply, neighboring organs, diaphragm, and viscera. Keep in mind that each intercostal space has its own intercostal nerve that arises from the thoracic spine. Tension in a muscle could be caused by restricted blood flow that may also cause the nerve to activate or become irritated. For all of these reasons, movements need to be included that open the space between the individual ribs in more than one direction. In general, it's a good idea to create and find movements that follow a variety of lines of action. We'll integrate these principles when we get into using the movements accompanying these anatomical perspectives.

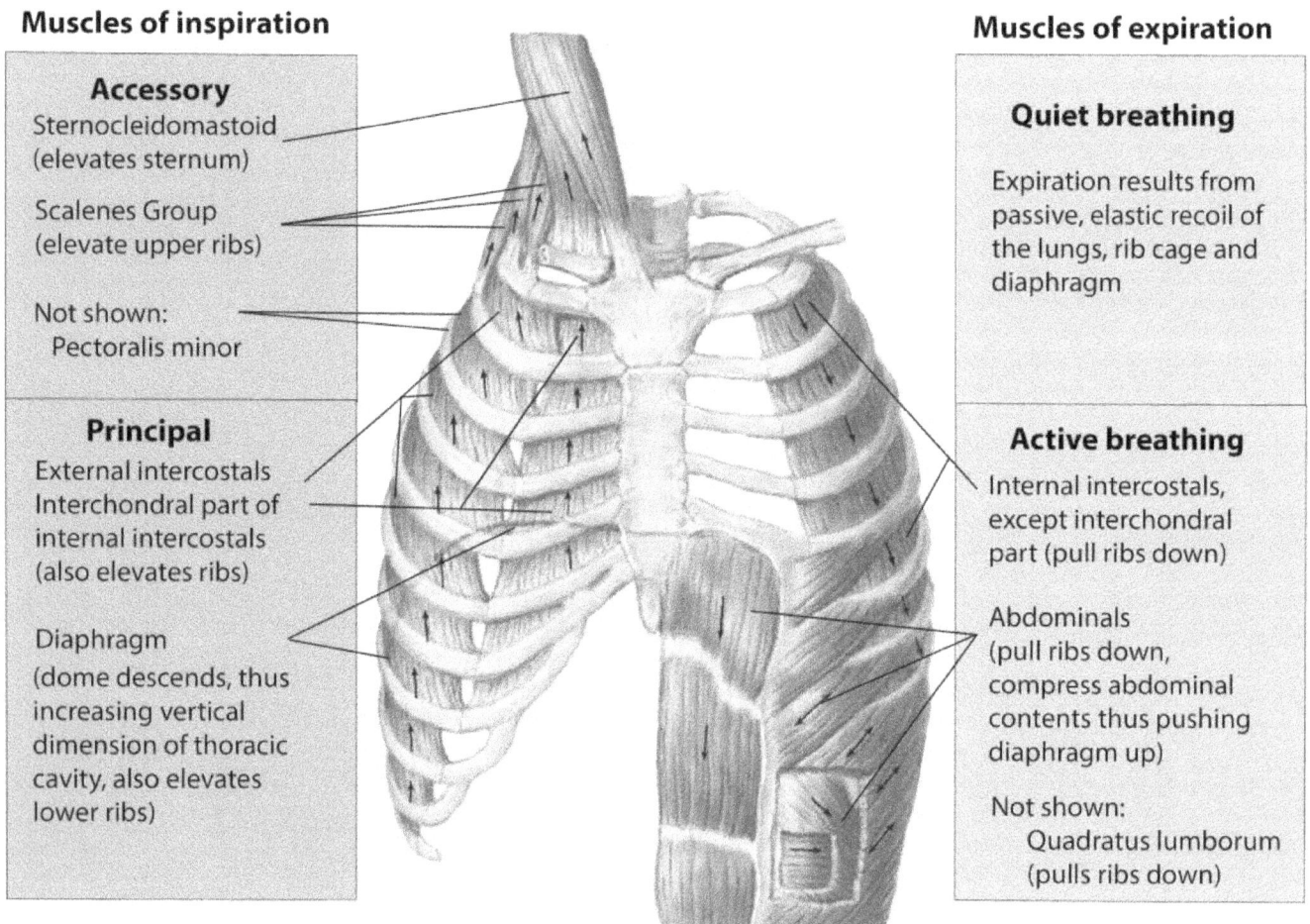

Muscles of inspiration

Accessory
Sternocleidomastoid (elevates sternum)

Scalenes Group (elevate upper ribs)

Not shown:
Pectoralis minor

Principal
External intercostals
Interchondral part of internal intercostals (also elevates ribs)

Diaphragm (dome descends, thus increasing vertical dimension of thoracic cavity, also elevates lower ribs)

Muscles of expiration

Quiet breathing

Expiration results from passive, elastic recoil of the lungs, rib cage and diaphragm

Active breathing

Internal intercostals, except interchondral part (pull ribs down)

Abdominals (pull ribs down, compress abdominal contents thus pushing diaphragm up)

Not shown:
Quadratus lumborum (pulls ribs down)

Fig. 1.14 – *Muscles of Respiration*
Courtesy of Netter and Elsevier via Wikimedia Commons

Tight chest muscles can mimic heart or lung issues. Shortness of breath, numbness down the arm, chest pain, or spasms can be caused by poor posture, poor digestion, a tight pectoralis minor or major, tight intercostal muscles, a subluxated rib, trigger points, and chest breathing. A seat belt injury, weightlifting, and contact sports that involve falling can contribute to muscle strain and tightness in the chest that can eventually restrict breathing and potentially compromise heart or lung function if left untreated. That said, it is clearly important to investigate each possibility, and make efforts to keep those areas that affect the heart or lungs as relaxed and able to freely function as possible.

Most people aren't used to thinking that they can actually have an influence on internal organs and their surrounding tissue, so initial attempts may not be as tuned in as they would be after practice. Those with trained hands will easily feel down through the layers and discern varying degrees of tension in one area of the thorax versus another, be it the pericardium or the pleura, the diaphragm or the linea alba. Give yourself time to practice. Start by gradually increasing your pressure (still very light) while visualizing which layer you intend to contact, and wait a few seconds for the tissue to respond. Explore the area both when it feels good/normal, and when it doesn't so you have a working frame of reference.

People have been known to throw out a rib, strain or spasm muscles, and even bulge a disc from a fit of coughing. Coughs are common with a cold or flu and can reach speeds between 50 and 100 mph, while a sneeze is much less at up to 35 mph. Those who have lingering coughing spells from pneumonia or other conditions can accumulate tensions in the thorax, in between ribs, and in the abdominal, back, and groin areas. It's easy to forget what caused the strain in these instances because those tensions don't automatically leave your system. It's helpful to have a few movements you can do on your own to release and rebalance these tissues of the thorax and alleviate additional pressure on the heart and lungs, including the protective membranes (Fig. 1.15).

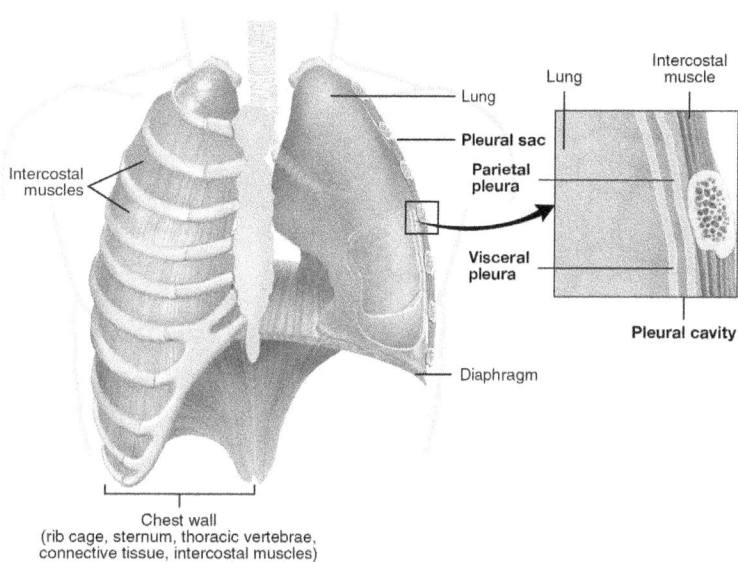

Fig. 1.15 - *Internal membranous layers of the chest wall including the diaphragm and its attachments. (Not shown - linea alba beneath the xyphoid process)*
Image courtesy of OpenStax College, CC BY 3.0 via Wikimedia Commons

Due to the sheer numbers of people around the world who are affected by issues with this vital organ that has limited abilities to replenish itself structurally, it is much more important to understand what influences its well-being. All ages are affected by heart issues, and although exercise can be a great help, it can also remodel the heart in ways that increase risk. The first exercises illustrated here will address ways to open the space around the heart and lungs as well as to facilitate breathing. In keeping with the embryological perspective, we will begin by addressing the heart through the midline.

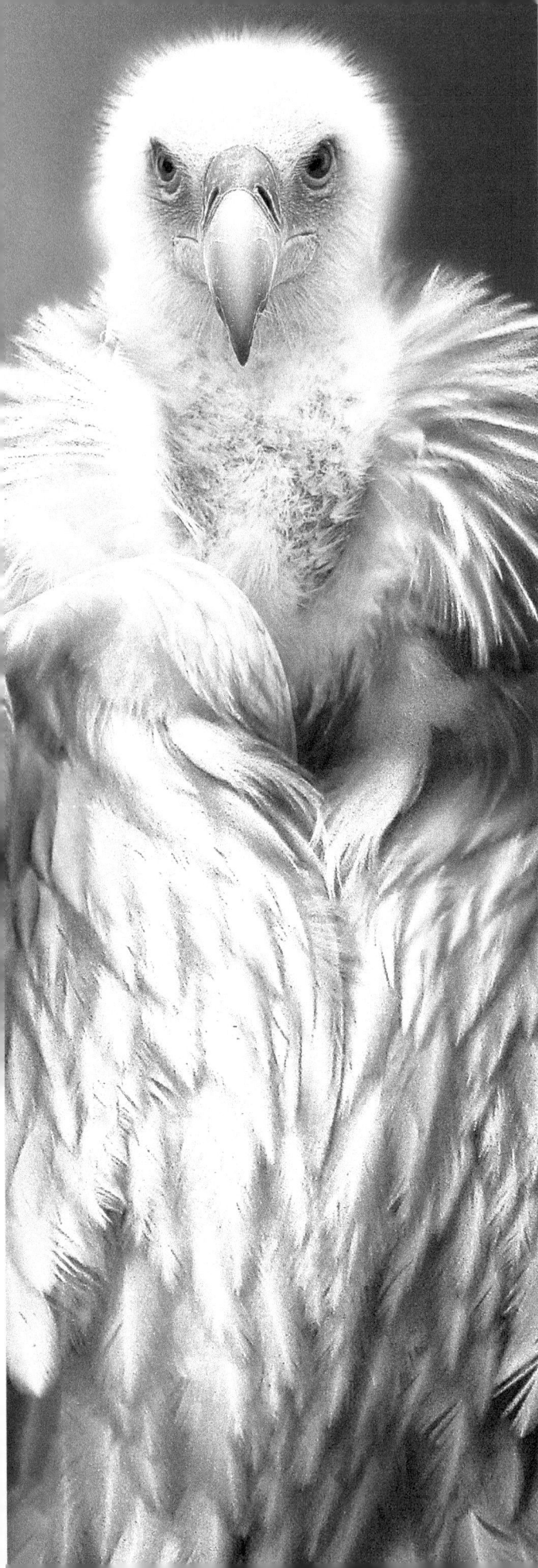

Chapter 2
Getting a Sense of Things

The midline is the root

Life begins at the midline of our bodies. An enormous amount of information passes through the branches of the root to sustain the body's needs in a balanced, efficient way. Much of the regulatory processing for the internal glands, musculoskeletal system, and organs happens via the brain and nervous system's interactions with them. Many of the details about exactly how that happens and why these core structures remain key signaling and processing centers throughout life is discussed in Volume 8 of the Somatic Intelligence series: Movement is Medicine.

This volume will focus on a variety of movements that help free the structures along the midline/root, including the spine, heart, blood and other fluid systems, muscles and connective tissue, as well as the nervous system. All of these systems also participate in the energetic channels and centers being able to function without restriction. Before we dive into the movement series, it would be most helpful for the long-term goal of becoming self-regulatory if you become more aware of exactly what you're moving, and learn to sense into this anatomy and "listen" for feedback from it.

The midline and movement

There are nerve roots that exit vertebral segments and connect to the function of all of our muscles. (Fig. 2.1) Decompressing and aligning these segments can help those muscles to settle down and relax, and vice versa. The **phrenic nerve**, which originates from cervical vertebral segments C3, C4, and C5, passes through the thoracic inlet under the clavicle and along either side of the pericardial sac before inserting into and innervating the diaphragm. As we learned in the first chapter, the diaphragm is a very important muscle. A wide variety of daily life activities and experiences can elevate, maintain, or detract from the effectiveness of regulatory functions.

The initial movement sequences here will suggest where to place your attention and how to build awareness of sensations in the body. These sensations will become your guideposts for remaining in neutral balance and for avoiding or recovering from injury, stress, or strain. In every case, it's good to treat your body like a sensitive, intelligent, responsive organism that you're introducing yourself to in order to build a lasting relationship.

The **subcortical** system—or the autopilot mode—contains learned responses that are already filed and can fire in milliseconds. What you'll experience with conscious touch is different. Your body will be listening to every move you make and sending feedback, but it may be slower than you're used to. Similar to the times we want to change something in our behavior, we need to slow down, bring awareness in, and consciously choose the newer, preferred behavior. The body is the same way.

The conscious/**cortical** system in the "head" brain is where the "magic" happens. This is where cellular signaling systems from all over the body interact with the brain to review experiences and bring past knowledge and current intention to the choice point. As you learn to pause and feel for how the tissue responds when you change something even a little bit, you may be pleasantly surprised at how dynamic the experience is. Many aches and pains will fade as the body uses its own language to express its new status based upon **your intention, manual input, and clarifying movement.** You will get better and better at deciphering those messages.

We're trained not to "baby" ourselves, but it's far better to take note of the initial signal the body sends out to let you know something's uncomfortable than to wait until it becomes painful. The body will revert to auto-pilot mode, perhaps grasping at straws to compensate, until it receives current updates in the form of conscious input from you. We are a key contributor within the sensory-motor feedback loop as a part of the system's ongoing conversation with itself, as are daily life stressors and cumulative tension.

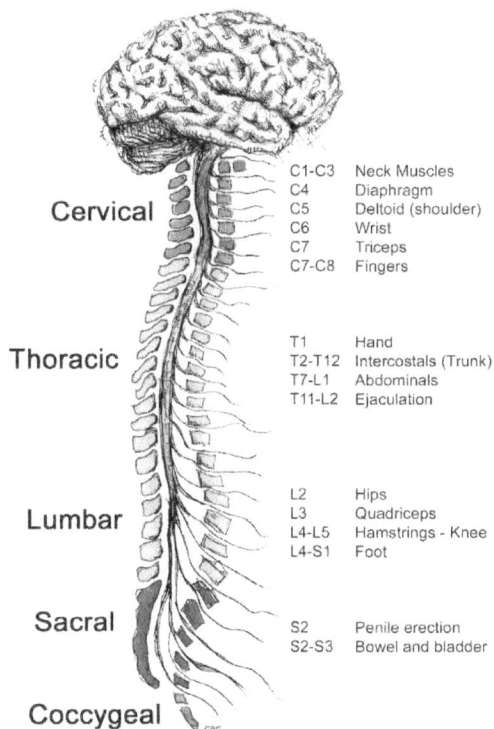

	C1-C3	Neck Muscles
	C4	Diaphragm
Cervical	C5	Deltoid (shoulder)
	C6	Wrist
	C7	Triceps
	C7-C8	Fingers
	T1	Hand
Thoracic	T2-T12	Intercostals (Trunk)
	T7-L1	Abdominals
	T11-L2	Ejaculation
	L2	Hips
	L3	Quadriceps
Lumbar	L4-L5	Hamstrings - Knee
	L4-S1	Foot
Sacral	S2	Penile erection
	S2-S3	Bowel and bladder
Coccygeal		

Fig. 2.1 – *Diagram of spinal nerves and what they innervate. They can easily be affected by posture and use patterns.*
(Courtesy of Creative Commons)

It will facilitate much more cooperation and ease of release for the midline structures if the adjacent forces are released first. Consider that every move you make with the arms, legs, hips and shoulders, impacts the central structures. Many of those peripheral structures attach at or near central tissue fields and the spine itself, making the midline vulnerable to any imbalances that are in these adjacent fields of influence.

Using the **mechanotransduction system** located throughout all fascia, bone, fluids, skin, muscle, and its adjacent connective tissue, we will incorporate the fundamental component of awareness to generate global, changes by awakening these systems' ability to sense and execute what is needed. In the process, you will also be awakening to the ways in which the system compromised its ability to move freely. By unconsciously grasping at straws, it created patterns that were a stop-gap measure at the time, then became imbedded by repetition in ways that were imbalancing. Your conscious participation will help prevent those patterns from becoming reinstalled or reinforced, and quickly free your system from stiffness, tension, aches, pains, and all sorts of discomfort or dis-ease.

Everywhere in the system, the ways by which the body transduces mechanical into chemical information is complex and largely conserved since its embryological origins. The endoderm, related to internal organs and the processing of food for the fetus, happens immediately after the formation of the ectoderm (skin) and nervous system. We can see how, in the adult body, the nervous system is still intimately related if not regulated by the nerves for sensory feedback and muscle function.

The core midline structures that are vital for life rely upon input from outside itself to satisy its basic needs, and they rely upon us to decode that input and keep its flow of critical feedback unimpeded. Just like in the wild, it's actually a matter of life or death, and also a matter of quality of life. In this book the focus will be on how to move in a way that matters to maintaining both the vital aspects of life, in addition to the more nuanced aspects of genuine, blissful well-being.

We will begin the process by releasing many of the peripheral forces that apply restrictions and pressures to the midline's fundamental neutral balance before learning movements. The underlying principle here, is that a healthy core is not separate from emotional, mental, energetic, and spiritual health, each of which can also be mitigated by movement and manual therapies. Let's start with the basic foundation that supports the rest—the organization of the skeleton in relation to the spine.

Factors in unlearning and reorganizing posture

There are several contributors to how our posture becomes formed. Congenital defects aside, all of them are learned. Adolescence is a key period when growth and hormonal spurts happen, both of which can have an influence. Personality is a big factor, as it influences whether a pattern of withdrawal and shyness, or approach and outgoing assertiveness will predominate. Participation in sports, dance, gymnastics, and other athletic pursuits can also have a strong influence on the shape of the musculoskeletal system. Personal history as far as accidents, illnesses, or surgeries are potential factors.

Common postural adaptations

As you can see, most likely all of these subjects in the example are under 25 years- old, yet patterns have already been clearly established. (Fig.2.2) All but one have varying degrees of a forward neck, two have an exaggerated lordotic curve in the lower back, and one has a posterior (tucked) rotation of the pelvis. One has the kyphotic curve exemplified in the uupper thoracic spine, which creates a bit of a sunken chest. Not everyone has the same skeleton, and not every skeleton will be symmetrical, so we're not trying to fit a mold.

What seems like slight changes in how a person sits or stands can increase the pounds of pressure on a joint or disc by quite a bit (Fig.2.1). Any change in intervertevral disc height could affect nerve roots, innervation of muscles, and consequential tensions that tend to accumulate. Mostly every client I've spoken to about this issue is aware that their posture is off and that working at a desk or standing at a computer has had a huge impact on how they feel. Most are not aware of how to change it so that it's more balanced without tremendous muscular effort, which winds up being tiring. The methods you're about to learn will not need muscle power to attain the result we're looking for.

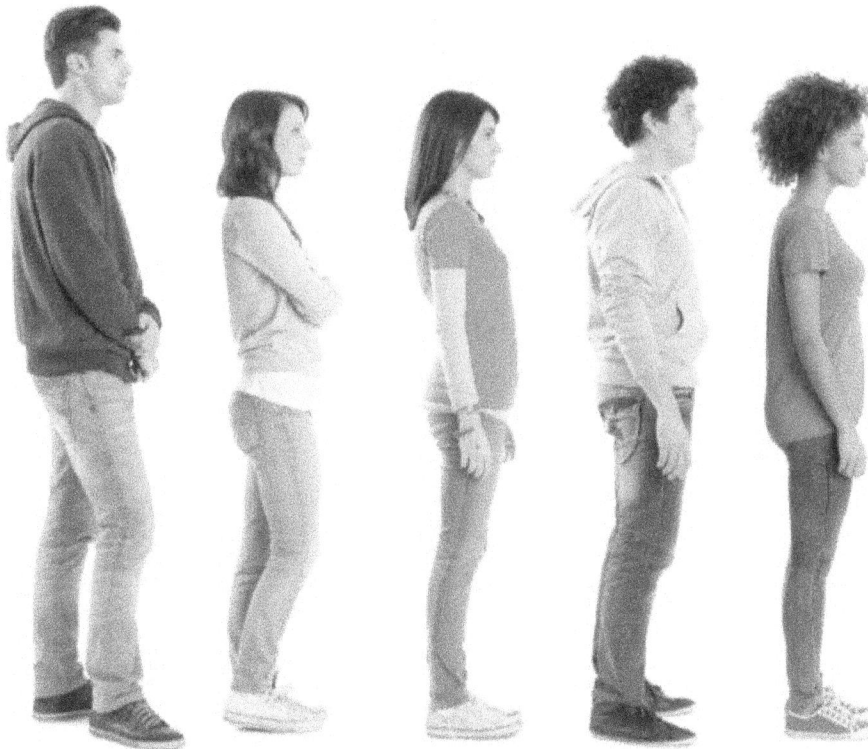

Fig. 2.2 – *Examples of mild posture modifications*

Section 1

Exploring Sensory and Somatic Awareness While Standing

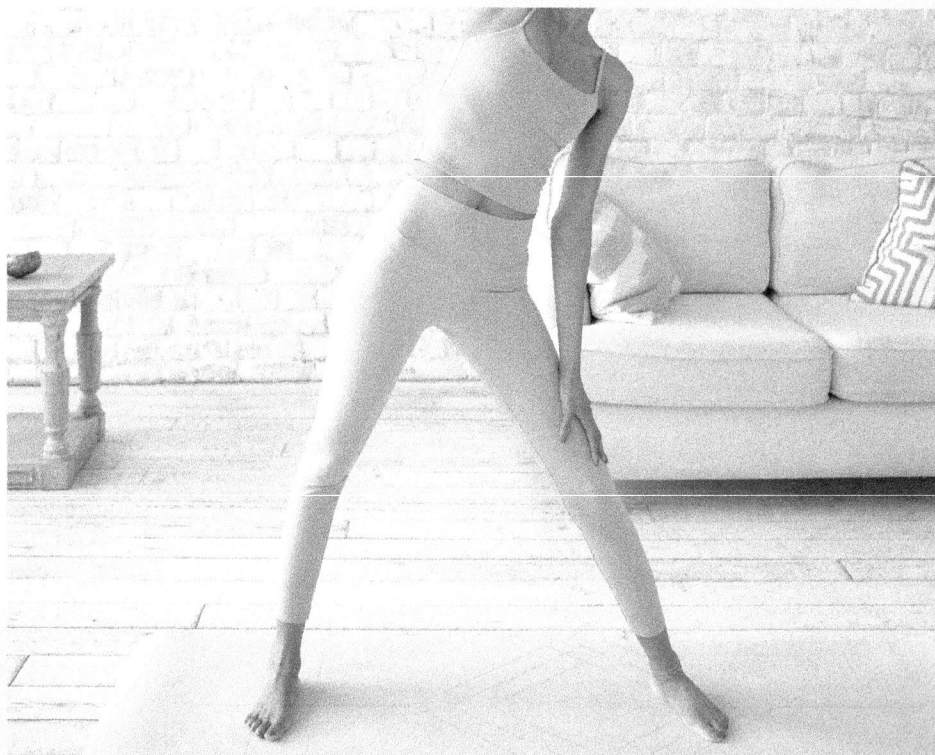

> Everything that happens to us in our lives causes a necessary reaction in our nervous system. Our brain responds and adapts to the events that occur. If we suffer shocks, accidental injury, serious illness, or complex surgery, our brain adapts to it. These are the events that bring on sensory-motor amnesia.
>
> — **Dr. Tom Hanna**

It's important to find neutral balance using structural references first, but later on you'll be able to use sensory information to correct the alignment. Achieving balanced posture in sitting or standing using sensory information is described in detail in Volume 7 of this series, You Are the Fulcrum, but it will be covered here in a more traditional way. If at all you're not certain using either frame of reference, you can always look in a mirror to see if your felt-sense matches what you see. The main frame of reference, optimally, will be your body's effortless ease.

Although we'll address a bit of the anatomical, biomechanical and biochemical factors initially, where we're headed is into the sensorium where the existential joy of being embodied lives. There, the interconnections between and within systems also become more and more apparent and shift before your body's "inner eyes," also known as its **interoceptive** system. This system is in the parietal lobe of the brain and uses proprioceptors to sense or perceive where its parts are in relation to the whole, and to the other parts. We will rely on this sense constantly as it awakens during this process.

As we approach health based upon neutral posture in this volume, we'll use the midline and its embryologically significant structures and related energetic pathways as the basis. Using this approach means establishing clear communication through tissue fields to accomplish wanted changes. It facilitates the natural, swift transmission of the necessary input because the body is designed to pay attention to the function of these structures. A key point here, is that optimum structural organization is inextricable from optimum functioning. Optimum functioning happens with clear communication throughout the system, and the best forms of communication are most likely the ones the system used when the body was being created: ectoderm, endoderm, mesoderm, at the midline.

Vertebral column disorders

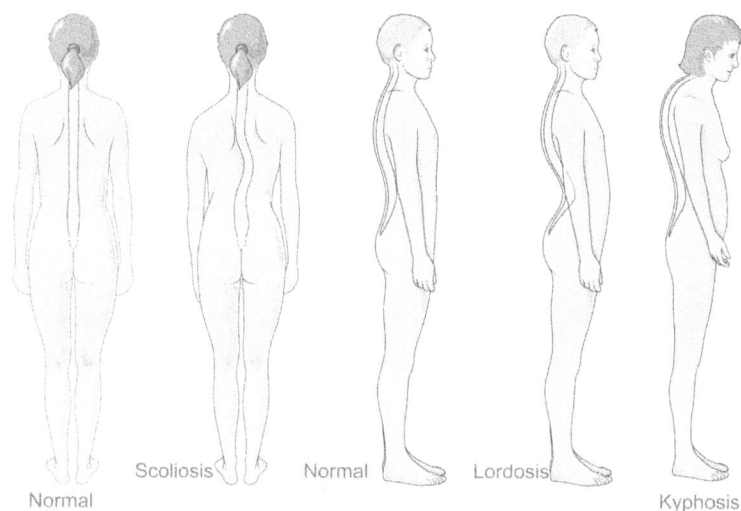

Normal   Scoliosis   Normal   Lordosis   Kyphosis

Fig. 2.3 – *Examples of postural distortions*

Being out of alignment means the muscles will have to work harder to keep you up at an angle that distorts or impedes the flow of input, energy, nutrients, and expulsion of waste. It will also cause compensatory reactions throughout the system. As you may have noticed from Fig. 2.1, several muscles and internal organs are connected to the nerves that exit each spinal segment, so it can be significantly beneficial to keep postural adaptations to a minimum (Fig. 2.3).

Most distortions can be corrected as they are functional, based on use patterns, rather than being congenital. However, as you saw in Figure 2.2, distortions can happen at a very young age, and they will begin to influence internal organs, the viscera, nerve function, mood, muscle tone, and overall health. Posture may not be among the initial recommendations to consider in order to resolve the issues unless the connections are already established in your mind.

Text Neck

In recent years, there has been another factor that greatly influences posture and strains the spine: time spent on cell phones and tablets (Fig.2.4). The additional weight that this altered position in gravity applies to the spine is considerable. It wouldn't be unusual for the kyphotic reaction at the upper thoracic spine to develop as a way to provide more tissue support to bear the additional strain of being bent forward. It could also compromise discs or nerve pathways, and lead to pain, numbness, tingling, headaches, eye strain, and shoulder tension.

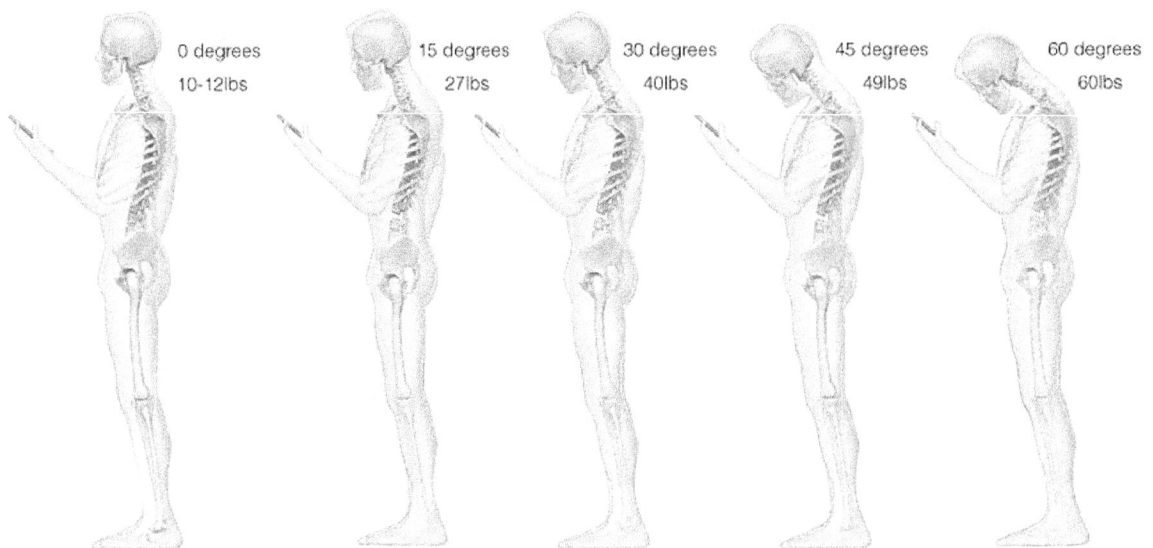

| 0 degrees | 15 degrees | 30 degrees | 45 degrees | 60 degrees |
| 10-12lbs | 27lbs | 40lbs | 49lbs | 60lbs |

Fig. 2.4 – Pounds of pressure added to the spine while the head and neck are in flexion from what is known as "text neck." The strain also happens while seated. Courtesy of Kenneth Hansraj, CC BY-SA 3.0 via Wikimedia Commons

The same issue could occur while reading a book or magazine when the tendency is to hold it on your lap. In fact, you can consider that any type of work or activity (like lab technicians peering through a microscope all day) can have a similar outcome. Some activities will prove to be difficult to adjust the position you're in, but as long as you're prepared to take care of those tensions as they arise, you'll be fine.

> *Most agree that the plumb line (Fig. 2.5) extends from the ear through the shoulder joint, the greater trochanter of the hip, the middle of the knee, and down through the ankle bone. There are natural cervical, thoracic, and lumbar curves that are useful and necessary for the spine to absorb and dissipate the forces coming up the legs while upright. Maintaining a posture that aligns with these landmarks is supposed to be the ideal way to receive gravitational forces.*

In general, the **plumb line** is still the best frame of reference for the posture the body needs to receive gravitational forces (Fig. 2.5).

Lateral View Markers

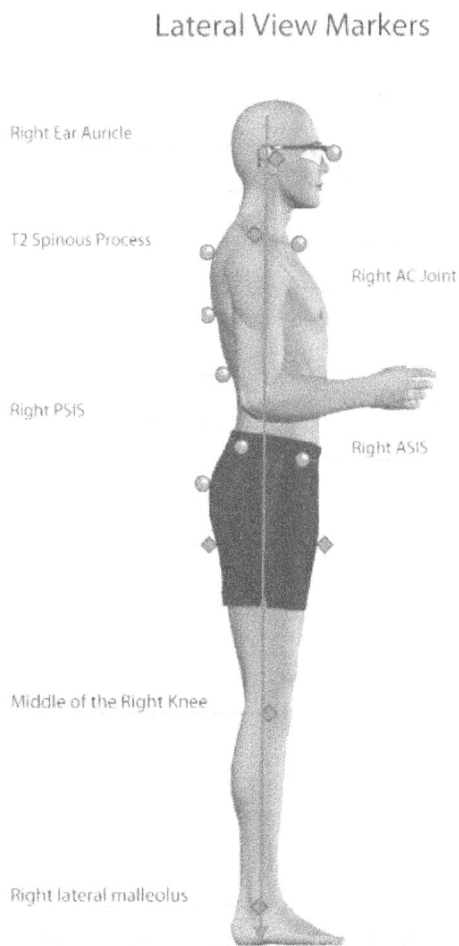

Right Ear Auricle

T2 Spinous Process

Right AC Joint

Right PSIS

Right ASIS

Middle of the Right Knee

Right lateral malleolus

Fig. 2.5 - The Plumb Line

Finding Your Plumb Line

Sensing Posture Exercise #1

Take a moment to sense those areas in your own spine, and feel whether you can distinguish between the thoracic curve and the lumbar curve. Then notice the cervical curve and whether the soft tissue on one side of the spine feels different in any way than on the other side of the spine for each area: cervical, thoracic, and lumbar.

Sensing Posture Exercise #2

Shift your awareness to the anterior of your body while maintaining attention at the thoracic spine curvature. Get a sense of the bony feel of the sternum (center of the ribs), and of the space filling the cavity itself where your heart and lungs are.

Sensing Posture Exercise #3

Close your eyes and tune into the spine and ribs in the back and the sternum and ribs in the front. Notice how they move when you breathe. Do the same for the organs in the thorax. In which directions do the ribs move with ease?

Sensing the body cavity exercises

If you are already involved with conscious movement or hands-on practices, you may be able to feel the subtle motion of the organs and fluids. If you do, make note of the rate or pace of their motion and compare it to other days or activities to see if your rhythm changes. How does your breath feel? Does it change when you breathe into your chest rather than into your belly? Is it full or shallow, more forceful on the inhale or during the exhale? Do your ribs or clavicles move?

Sensing the thorax - feel what's inside the space

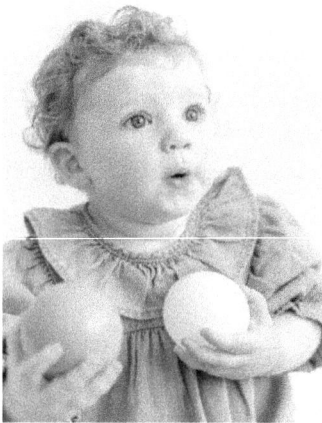

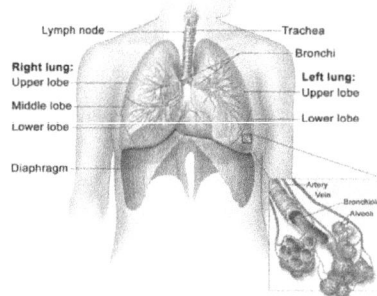

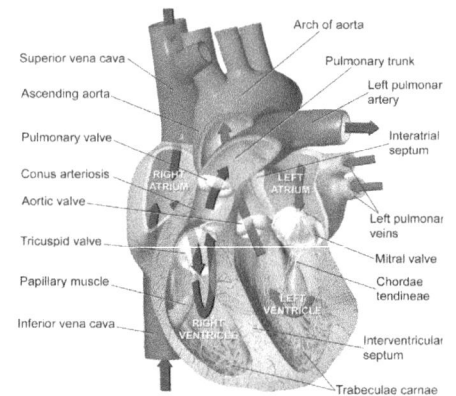

Sectional Anatomy of the Heart

Fig. 2.6 – *Interior of the lungs*   **Fig. 2.7** – *Interior of the heart*

Let yourself return to the newness and curiosity that is prevalent in the life and mind of a child. Take a moment to sense the front, back, and sides of your chest, as though you were holding a large ball and noticing the dimensions of it, both outside and inside, for the first time. Where does it feel bouncier and more elastic on your ribs versus more stiff and rigid? Where does it feel more open and spacious versus more solid? Can you feel your heart beating stronger in one area than another? The lungs seem to be spacious, but they are filled with bronchioles and blood vessels (Fig. 2.6). The heartbeat can be felt in every artery in the body. The heart has more space in its chambers, yet is semi-filled with blood (Fig. 2.7); can you sense any differences between the way the heart and lungs feel, in a very general way?

Does the tissue move underneath your hands? Very often the skin, muscles, and fascia will begin to shift as soon as there is contact, lending themselves to softening and opening. You may notice a change in direction, as one area begins to shift to the right, or downward, or even off at an angle. The body may immediately begin to self-correct into a more balanced organization with that little bit of conscious touch and self-sensing.

Sensing and comparing the thorax with the abdominal cavity

You can change the position of your hands to include a place that is lower in the thorax, where your liver, intestines, kidneys, pancreas, stomach, and spleen are (Fig. 2.8). Are you able to notice any difference between the feeling of the stomach, which is a hollow organ, and the liver, which is not? The organs express a universal, rhythmic motion that is consistent and paired. The pancreas is so deep and wide that it crosses the midline and moves with the stomach and spleen rather than the liver on the right side. See if where you place your hands increases and facilitates motion, or whether it decreases and inhibits motion.

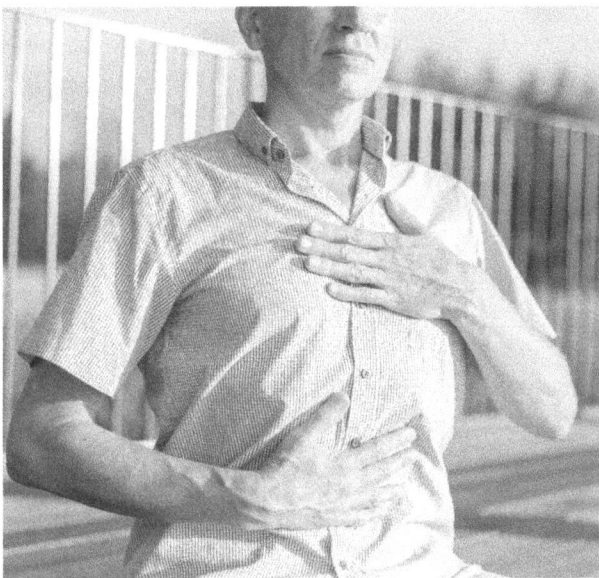

Feel and compare the qualities within the chest and abdomen

Internal organs

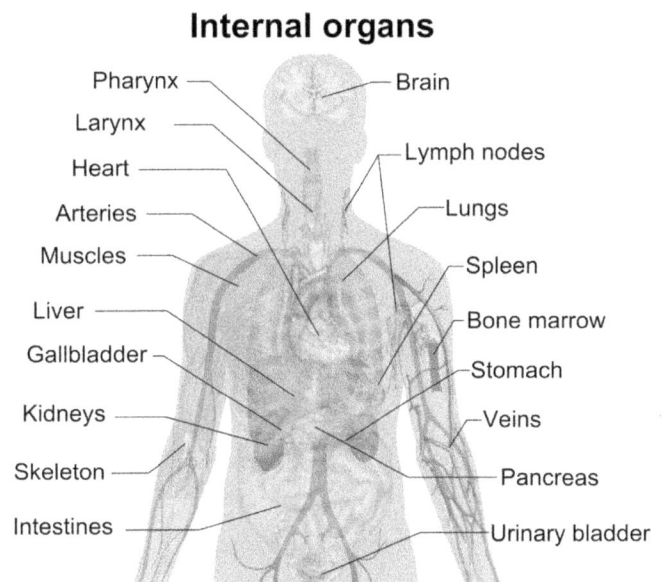

Pharynx

Larynx

Heart

Arteries

Muscles

Liver

Gallbladder

Kidneys

Skeleton

Intestines

Brain

Lymph nodes

Lungs

Spleen

Bone marrow

Stomach

Veins

Pancreas

Urinary bladder

Fig. 2.8 – *Internal organs within the chest and abdomen*

Sensing the body's response to your hands

If you place your hands directly on top of the small intestine, for example, as long as your contact is light, there will still be motion. If it's pressing in too much, things will likely slow down to a halt. Do the organs or viscera shift their position in reponse to your contact? Which direction is the shift? Which structure moved? Place your hand above the belly button and locate the soft tube running horizontally across the space (transverse colon) (Fig. 2.9). Did it gurgle? Follow it around where it becomes the descending colon, then the sigmoid colon, which lies on top of the iliacus on the left side.

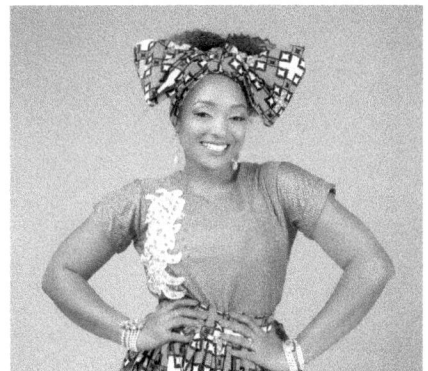

This can easily become a sticking point for the iliopsoas and the colon. See if you can get in between the inner rim of the ilium and the soft, round tube and very gently, slowly press in, away from the rim of the ilium. Your breath will improve immediately because the surrounding membranes of the thorax and abdomen are interconnected. Females have a few horizontal structures in the pelvic cavity (the broad, cardinal, and cervical ligaments) that may relax and open when you place your hands consciously on your hips and gently press in.

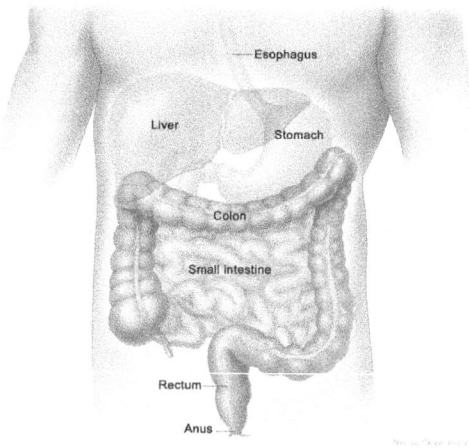

Fig. 2.9

Courtesy of Blausen.com staff (2014). "Medical gallery of Blausen Medical 2014." WikiJournal of Medicine 1(2)DOI:10. 15347/w/m/2014 010. ISSN 2002-4436, CC BY-SA 3.0 via Wikimedia Commons

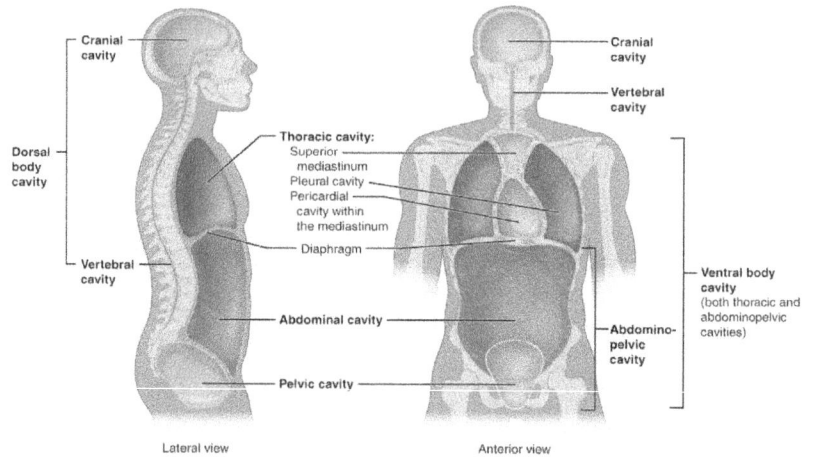

Fig. 2.10 – Illustration of Body Cavities
Courtesy of Connexions , CC BY SA 3.0, via Wikimedia Commons

The seemingly individual cavities (Fig. 2.10) and the organs or viscera within them are connected by the parietal peritoneum, which splits off to surround each individual organ (Fig. 2.11), with the exception of the kidneys. If you're near the last rib, you may feel the gentle movement of your kidneys, which move in toward, and then out and away from one another. They're often described as feeling as slippery as a wet bar of soap. They're quite deep from the front, as they are just in front of the quadratus lumborum on the other side of the body. And they are retro-peritoneal, which means they are outside of the abdominal wall/parietal peritoneum.

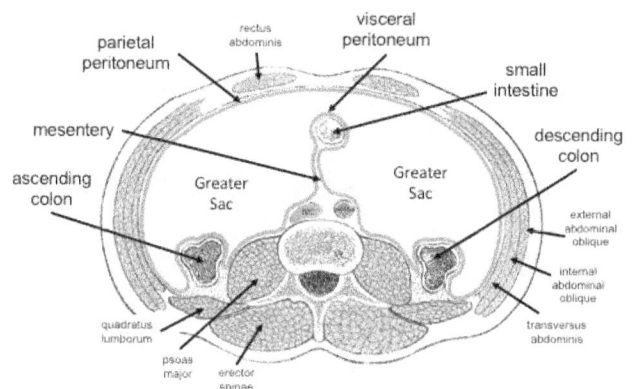

Fig. 2.11 - *Illustration of Parietal and Visceral Peritoneum in a cross-section view from above.*
Courtesy of Dennis M. DePace, PhD, CC BY-SA 4.0, via Wikimedia Commons

There are times that tension in the psoas muscle or in the quadratus lumborum will inhibit the smooth glide of the kidneys, so that's a good hint where to open things up if the kidneys aren't moving well. When your hands are further out and directly on top of the iliac crest of the pelvis, you might be able to notice whether one hand seems lower than the other, which is often the case. It is easily corrected. Check and see if you can feel the gentle pulsation of the femoral artery, which is just beneath the inguinal ligament. The flow is often impeded by the hours of sitting a person might be doing during the day or by other daily life tensions, surgeries, or accidents. These simple self-sensing exercises can give clues as to which movements to include in your routine, including how to open this vulnerable area.

Sensing through tissue layers using the skin as a signal transducer

1 - Sensing the skin and upper cavity

One very simple way to check the connectivity of the membranous layers just beneath the skin is to apply light pressure and gently press the skin front to back toward your spine. Notice the changes all around your back, ribs, and inside your chest. Notice how the tissue then gathers up around the neck and shoulders. Can you sense a little bit of compression around the liver, stomach, and lungs? Did the area around your lower back and sacrum decompress a little?

2 - Sensing changes by adding breath

Take a couple of deep breaths, first holding the inhale for 3 seconds, then the exhale. Watch how the layers of tissue, as well as the structures inside the thorax, and abdominal cacities respond to the light stretch from within combined with the activation of the breath. Notice whether your body opens more to the stretch or to the breath.

3 – Sensing the skin and lower cavities

Next, change the direction and lightly press down toward your feet, pressing in a little deeper than surface layers of skin. Without forcing, keep pressing in and down until the tissue provides a natural place to stop. Is there equal ease on the left side as there is on the right? Are there areas of tissue that release more easily in this direction than toward the head? Which direction is most affected by the breath?

4 - Creating changes by connecting cavities

Repeat this practice while changing the position of your hands higher, lower, more posterior, anterior or medially (in toward your navel). Return to specific areas in each cavity you noticed earlier to be stiffer. Combine a tense area in one cavity with a stiff area in another. When you feel the tissue begin to soften and lengthen under your hands, add your breath and wait for it to release all the way before exploring new combinations.

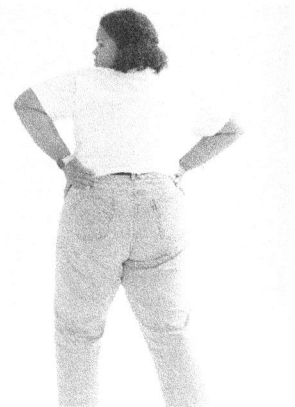

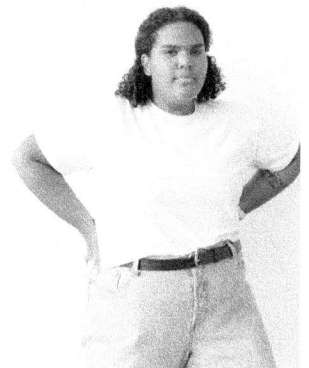

First your hands are on your hips, slowly press in until you can feel the shape of the pelvic bone without needing to touch it directly.

ONE SKY

5 – Adding movement as a way to wake up the brain

What enhances this potential for creating change even more is adding a movement involving the muscles while holding the stretch with the skin. Explore this phenomenon by taking a small step while pulling up on the tissue over the gluteal muscles and iliotibial tract. There will be a wonderful response down the side of the leg that rivals using a foam roller. This is true for any area that you use this method with. You can also rotate the leg in or out, move it further away from the other leg, and so on, to discover which aspect of the fascial chain is open to more opening and releasing. Try moving the skin sideways with the inhale and vertically with the exhale.

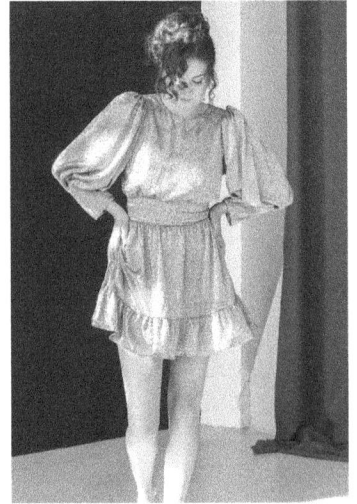

6 – Integrating cavity changes across trajectories

Up to now we've tried a variety of hand positions, but only used them with movements that are superior or inferior in direction (vertical). This time, explore moving the skin in a variety of angles. Try dragging it in a horizontal or diagonal direction within the same cavity or in combining different cavities. If an area feels more stuck when you drag the skin, add the breath and/or movement and see what your body listens and responds to more. Then go vertical again and combine it with horizontal or diagonal motion of the skin to allow the deeper fascia to take advantage of the openings in the superficial membranes. Remember that the skin is the first layer of our bodies to develop as an embryo, and it has a powerful capacity to create global changes at a cellular level.

Significance of the center of gravity

I believe that it's important for people to be more aware of what you're touching when you make contact with your body, and of what is moving underneath the skin as you move. As you grow in this relationship with the intelligent entity that is your body, it grows in its relationship with you. Soon, you'll be in such synchrony with your system that you can put your hands on your hips and they will immediately begin to rebalance the muscles and connective tissue. That area between your navel and your low back is your center of gravity, which is a major point of organization for whatever movement you'll be making. It is also the support for actions using the extremities.

You can become as familiar with your inside characteristics as you do some things you're passionate about on the outside, like a sport. Athletes become familiar with every aspect of the sport they're interested in, such as a tennis or golf pro who has experimented with and become certain about which brand racquet or clubs is preferred, and which club for which shot, which

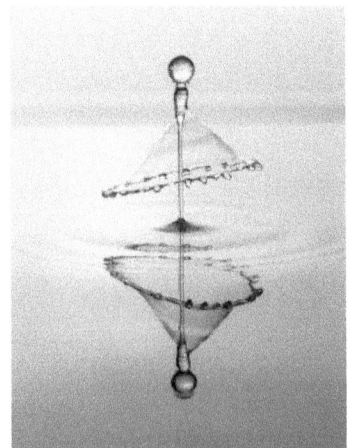

shoes, balls, and so on. Developing that type of relationship with your body where you've noticed and cared for all the details accordingly, will be just as rewarding as mastering an activity that you love. However, you can't go to any store and order a new body or a set of joints that will be as good as the originals, so it's even more important to remember what you notice and take good care.

If the bones are not balanced, the muscles will tighten, vessels will become restricted, efficiency of movement will be compromised, and energy will be diminished. As you can see, the sacrum doesn't look like the joints in the extremities, but it does have a slight bit of motion. Anyone who's had it badly out of alignment knows how awful it can feel. When the sides of the ilium rotate forward or back, get stuck up or down, or flare in or out, (Fig.2.15) it can also change the tone in the surrounding tissues and create discomfort. (Some people with these types of imbalance will not feel discomfort.) If you place your thumbs on the anterior superior iliac spine (ASIS) (Fig. 2.12) and look in the mirror, you will be able to compare the two sides and tell which type of imbalance is there, if any.

There are several nerve fibers and ligaments anterior to the sacrum that have an influence on how your lower back and central nervous system feel. You've seen in Figure 2.1 how the urogenital system is innervated by the nerves exiting the sacrum. In addition, there are numerous blood, nerve, and lymphatic vessels that run through this cavity that will react when the bones are off and the muscles tighten.

Very often, a level of tension or discomfort or loss of energy will be the sensations you feel before it becomes stiff, tight, and painful. Taking action on the first signs will generally prevent the later symptoms from arising. Before you begin stretching, check the bony landmarks for imbalances. Maintaining balance in the bones and soft tissues in the center of gravity (in front of the upper sacrum) supports the entire body and the flow of information from one end to the other.

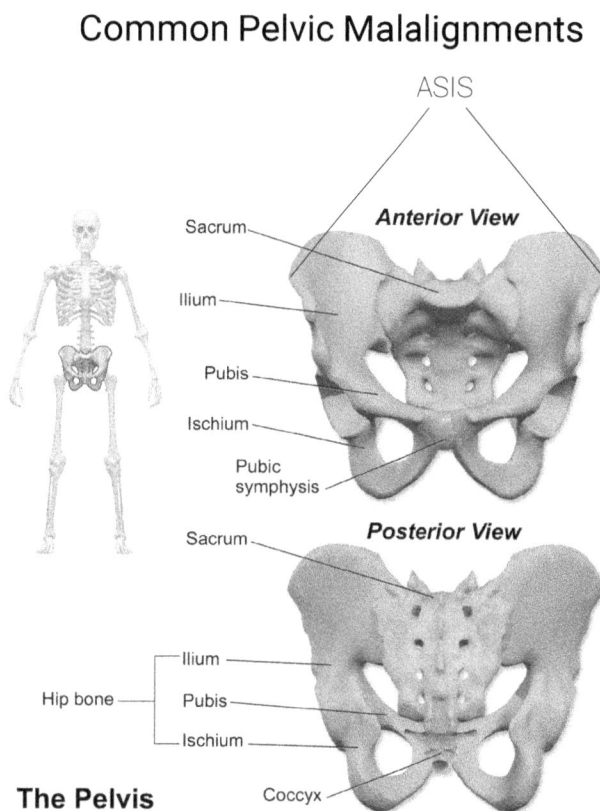

Common Pelvic Malalignments

ASIS

Sacrum
Ilium
Pubis
Ischium
Pubic symphysis

Anterior View

Sacrum
Ilium
Hip bone — Pubis
Ischium
Coccyx

Posterior View

The Pelvis

Fig. 2.12 – *Bones of the pelvis*
Image courtesy of Creative Commons International 3.0 Unported

Anterior rotation of one ilium

Posterior rotation of one ilium

Anterior View

Sacrum
Ilium
Pubis
Ischium
Pubic symphysis

A

Upslip of one side of the pelvis

Downslip of one side of the pelvis

Anterior View

Sacrum
Ilium
Pubis
Ischium
Pubic symphysis

B

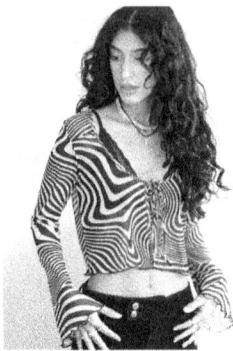

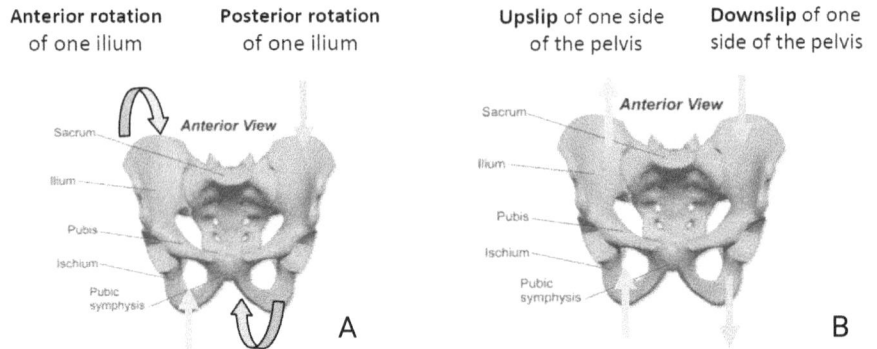

Fig. 2.13 - These are examples of the types of pelvic misalignments that can happen through use patterns or even while driving, particularly when there are bucket seats or a manual transmission. Uneven use of the legs while cycling or hiking can also produce a rotation as most people favor the dominant side. An **anterior or posterior rotation** involves one landmark being high, and the being low on that same side (A). In this case, the leg will appear short on that side. Landmarks may vary if the tibia or femur have been broken and reset in different lengths. An **upslip or downslip** (B) is less common, and involves one side with both landmarks being stuck either up or down after a fall or accidental force locks the muscles and bones in subluxation. Misalignments often happen in combination like an anterior rotation with a counter-rotation or outflare. In any case, you can learn to observe your bony landmarks and address the corresponding muscles. (See Chapter 3)

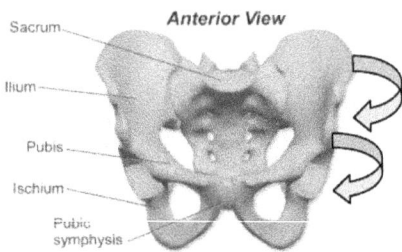

Anterior View

Sacrum
Ilium
Pubis
Ischium
Pubic symphysis

Fig. 2.14 – Example of a **Counter rotation** that often accompanies an anterior rotation of the right ilium while driving with one leg forward, whereby the entire pelvis has twisted to one side. Operating a sewing machine, surfing, fencing, boxing, or snowboarding are other activities during which it will be easy for the pelvis to twist like this.

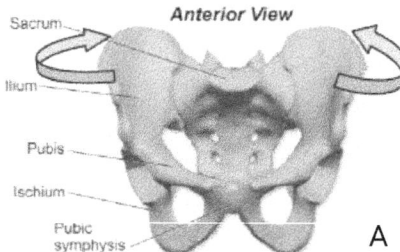

Anterior View

Sacrum
Ilium
Pubis
Ischium
Pubic symphysis

A

Fig. 2.15 – **Outflares (A)** are less common than inflares. **Inflares (B)** are often related to restricted blood flow, tight psoas or abdominal muscles, or internal organ issues.

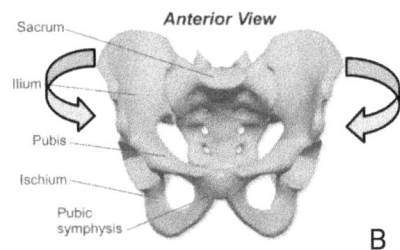

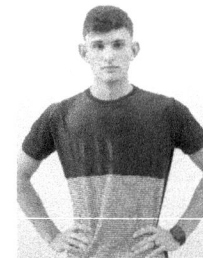

Anterior View

Sacrum
Ilium
Pubis
Ischium
Pubic symphysis

B

Males tend to have a narrower pelvis and are prone to inflares and outflares. Inguinal hernia surgery, soccer, and karate could produce an inflare or outflare. Males are also more vulnerable to inguinal hernias than women, so it's a good idea to keep this area balanced since 25% of those surgeries have complications,

Appreciating the importance and prevalence of fluids

It's good to be aware that whenever you're moving, it will be influencing fluid flow. It would be helpful to be aware of what and where these "rivers" are when you're in a particular position and notice whether you feel what we often call a "therapeutic pulse" as the area begins to open and allow more saturation of fluids. Fascia is drenched with fluid, bones and joints are filled with fluid, the brain is surrounded by and saturated with fluid, and even the Primo Vascular System contains fluid. They are great transporters of substances, signals, and information. The blood vessels in particular (Fig.2.16) can influence strength, temperature, and muscle tension anywhere in the body. What can seem like numbness from a restricted nerve can be caused by restricted blood flow.

Locating the major blood, nerve, and lymph vessels

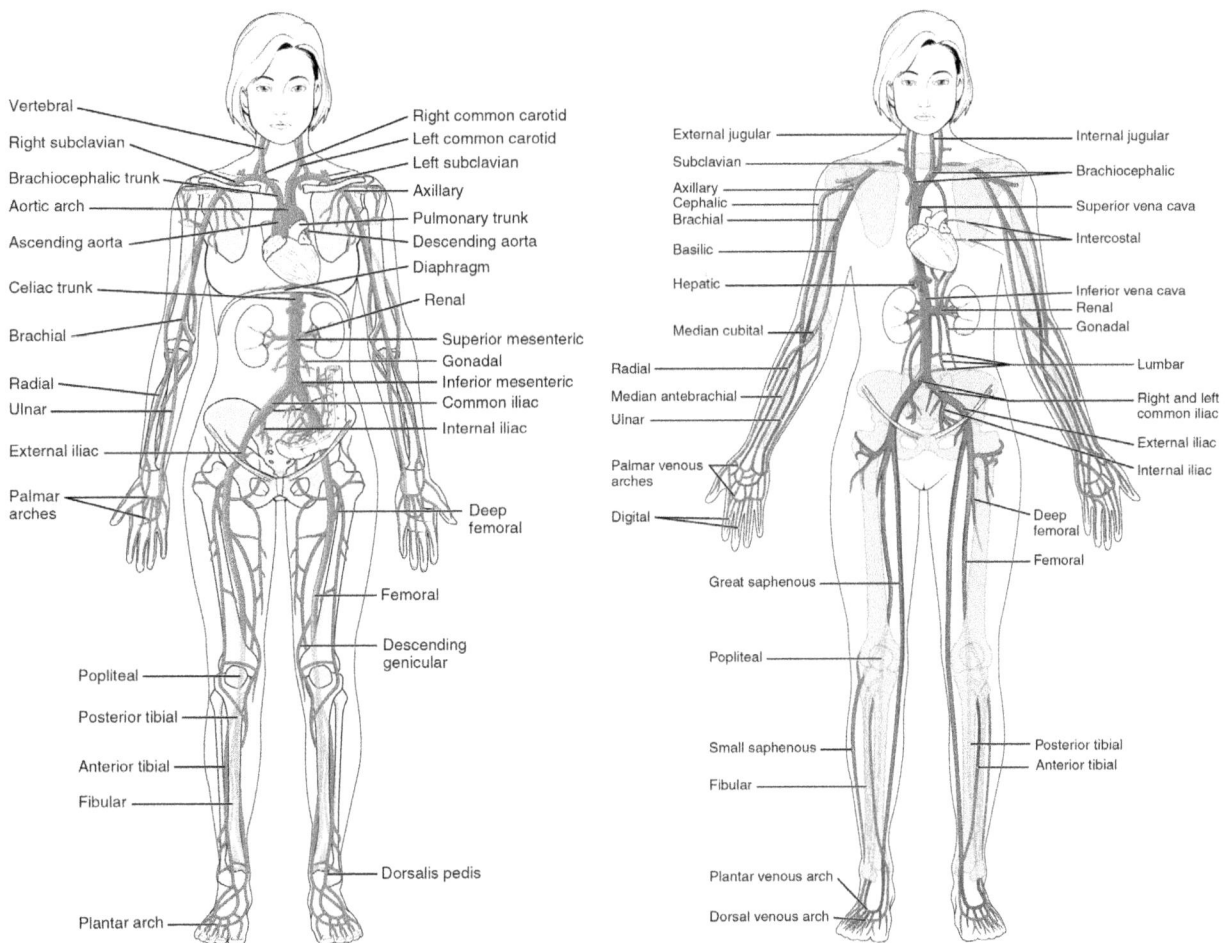

Fig. 2.16 - Major arteries and veins
Courtesy of OpenStax College, CC BY 3.0 via Wikimedia Commons

ONE SKY

You'll notice that the major vessels carrying blood throughout the body are prevalent in the midline and center of gravity, making posture all the more important to maintain. When the bones are aligned and blood and energy flow are unrestricted, nerve conduction (Fig. 2.17) and muscle tone will also be supported. The conduction of lymph fluids is also a key feature of maintaining health and muscle balance, and its unimpeded flow is dependent upon the circulatory system. Lymph vessels are practically everywhere in the body, although the ducts and nodes are in specific collections sites (Fig. 2.18).

Major nerves in the body

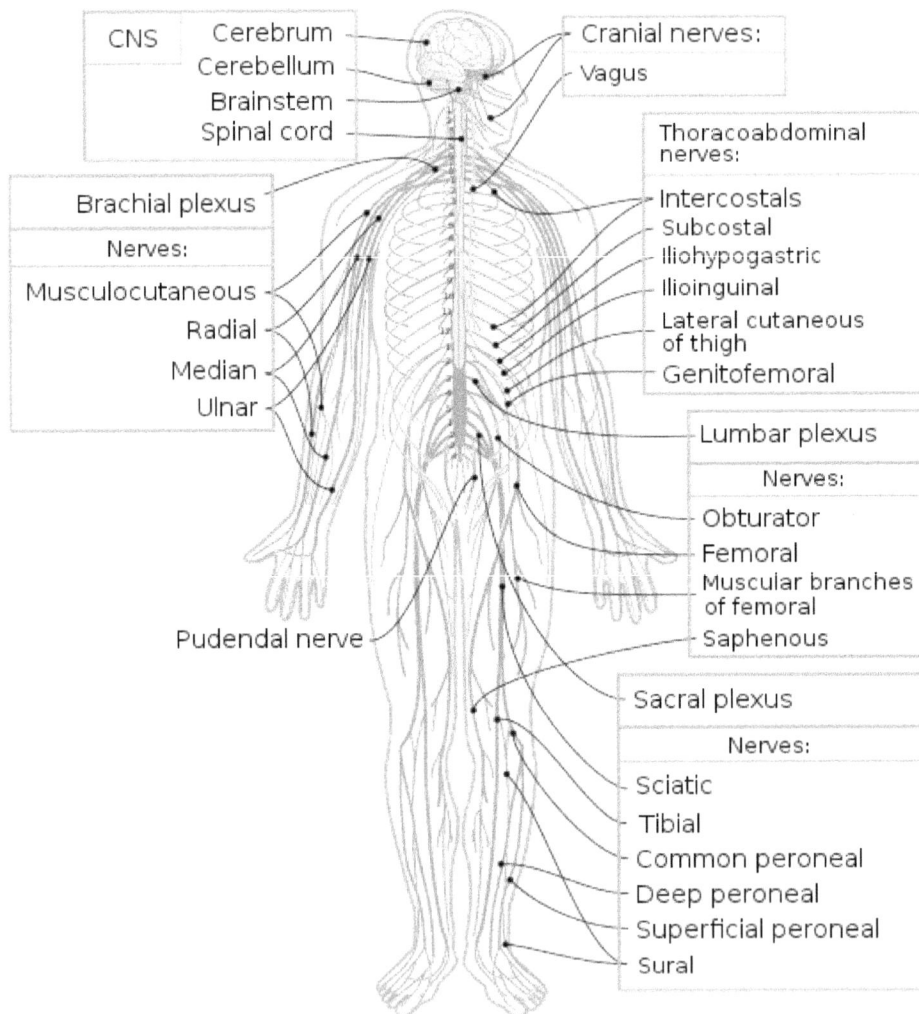

Fig. 2.17 – Major nerves in the body

Courtesy of Jmarchin, CC BY-SA4.0 via Wikimedia commons

Lymph vessels have a role in the body that revolves around maintaining fluid levels in the tissues and interstitial system by returning the plasma that seeps into the tissues from the capillaries back into the bloodstream (Fig. 2.19).

Lymph is largely composed of water, but there are also nutrients such as glucose, oxygen, amino acids, electrolytes, immunoglobulins, hormones, enzymes, vitamins, fats, and plasma proteins (i.e. albumin, fibrinogen, and globulin) that help maintain the colloidal osmotic pressure. The thoracic trunks—mostly the left one—drain the lymphatic capillaries back into the bloodstream.

Various lymph vessels, nodes, and ducts

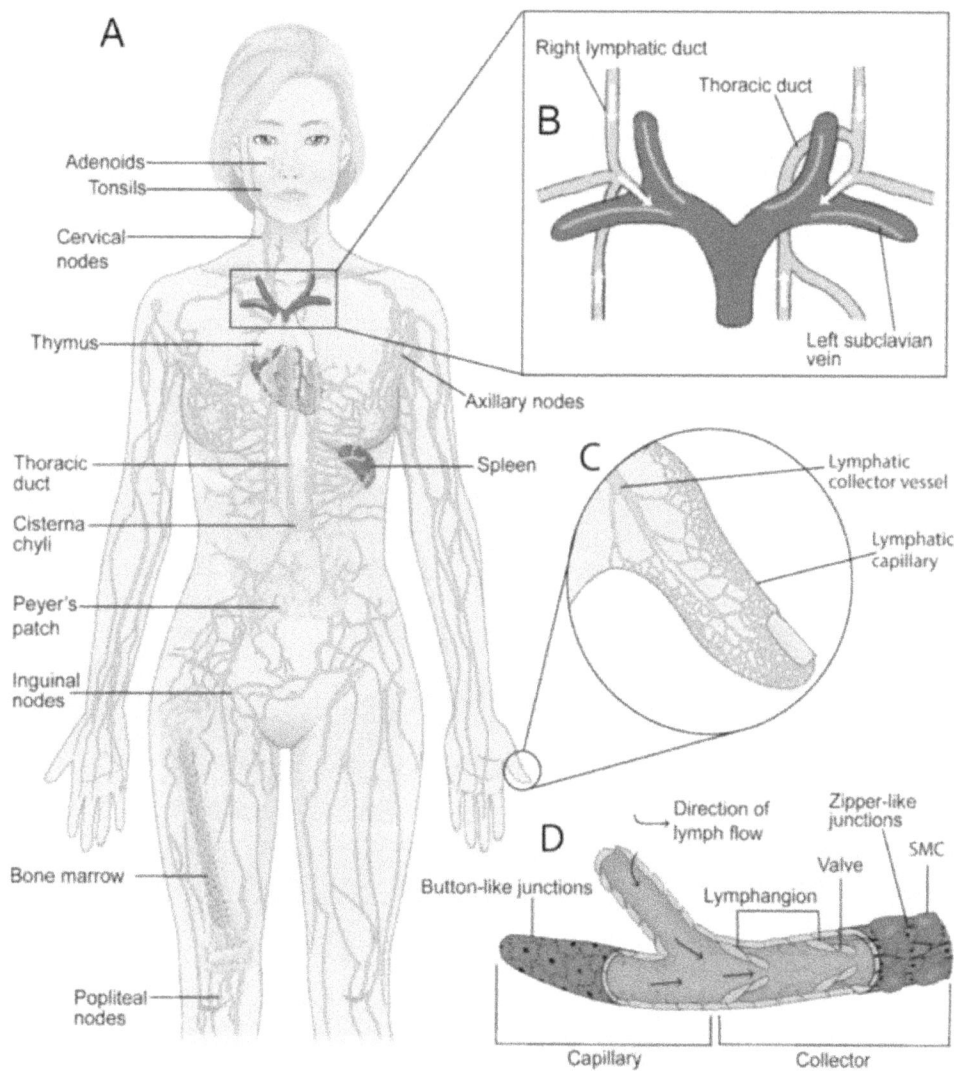

Fig. 2.18 – An illustration of the varied lymphatic anatomical components
Courtesy of OpenStax College, CC BY 3.0 via Wikimedia Commons

Lymph capillaries in the tissue spaces

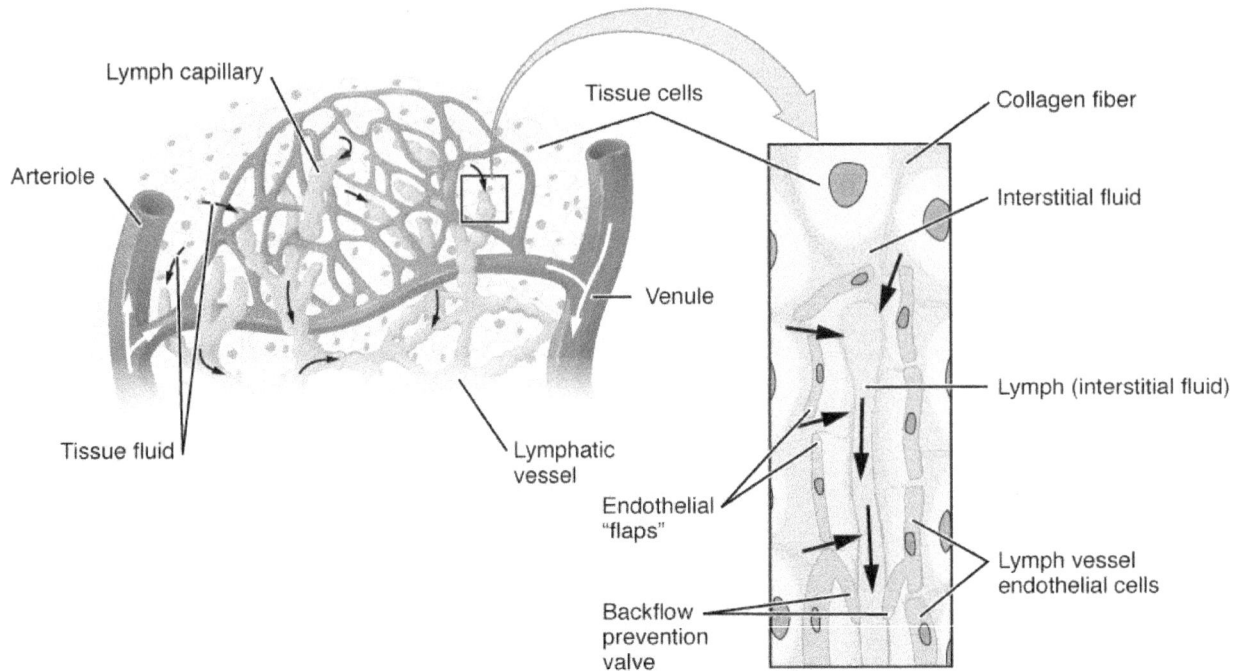

Fig. 2.19 – *Activity of the lymph capillaries between the tissue and interstitial spaces*
Courtesy of OpenStax College, CC BY 3.0, via Wikimedia College

If particulate matter or pathogens are present in the tissues or in interstitial fluid, they will be captured by the nodes and filtered. They will be prevented from entering the blood. The pathogens will be transported to the nodes where T-cell and B-cell lymphocytes in the white blood cells of the lymph will be activated and the pathogens are either being killed, metabolized, and/or neutralized by enzymes.

When antibodies are generated, the system will remember the pathogen and be protected in the future from it. Most people are familiar with the lymph nodes under the arms and in the groin area, as they are the ones that most frequently swell when some type of infection is present. Long hours sitting and/or wearing tight clothing could potentially limit the flow and activity of the lymph in these areas. You can make note that the cisterna chyli, that receives lymph fluids from the lower body and intestines, is in the midline. The fats from the intestines are distributed from here, and the lymph from the lower body is transported up the thoracic trunks that are also along the midline.

For many years, it was believed that jumping up and down was the only way to stimulate the lymph, and many people purchased trampolines during that time. We now believe that several different types of activities can facilitate lymphatic drainage, such as swimming, yoga, pilates, t'ai chi, hot and cold showers, drinking water, deep breathing, and workouts that tighten and pump the muscles. Manual lymph drainage can also be helpful. For serious lymph edema accompanying heart failure, for example, there are a few compression pumps for the extremities that are sometimes used.

Why to "end long" during your workouts

Keeping the concept of "pump" in mind, wherein the action involves an inward and outward flow, it's helpful to consider the outward flow. For the balance to be maintained, the same amount of fluid goes out as is coming in. This is a great frame of reference when using muscle groups during exercise, that you want the same amount of tension going out as is coming in. Although you may be gaining in strength, it's best to end long, as in using an eccentric rather than concentric contraction. In this way, if you've done several reps using moderate to heavy weights, you can discharge the strain that may have been accumulating in your neck, diaphragm, or in any of the critical midline structures. **For example:**

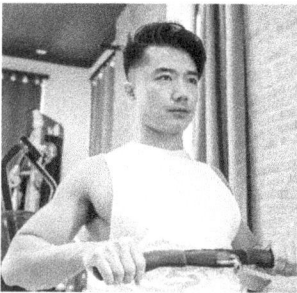

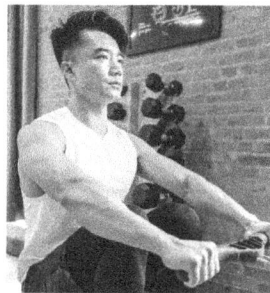

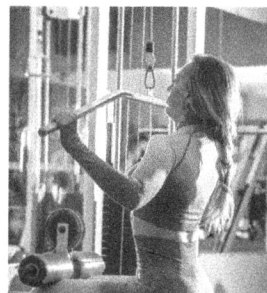

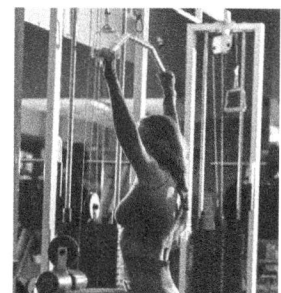

Whenever there's a machine or bar where you're doing pull-ups, lat pull-downs, or chin- ups, end long. Do the last couple of reps with a very gradual, conscious, gentle release into the full length of the muscles being used, with the arms fully extended. The same would hold true for sit-ups. Do the last couple by sitting back very slowly and flattening, then arching your back, head, and neck at the very end, extending everything you just flexed.

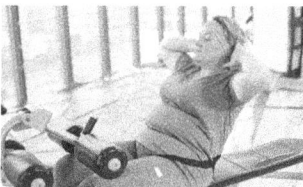

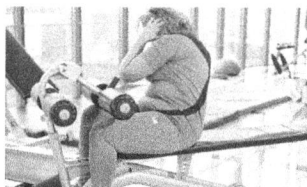

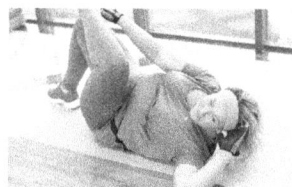

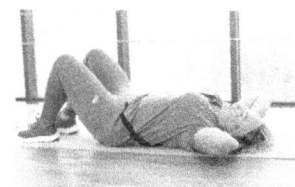

Each of these movements is able to pump the lymph. In the case of the woman above, because she's on a bench she could also extend her arms beyond the bench to get that extra opening across the chest, through the ribs, and into the diaphragm.

Make note of where the stomach, spleen, and liver are in relation to the diaphragm, all of which could lead to indigestion if their motion is compromised or if the stomach gets pushed up too high. After flexion exercises, it's best to at least flatten and if possible end with extension. This is a consideration for any exercise, particularly of the anaerobic type, which may serve to build muscle and pump the lymph, but can be even better for you with these few mindful adjustments.

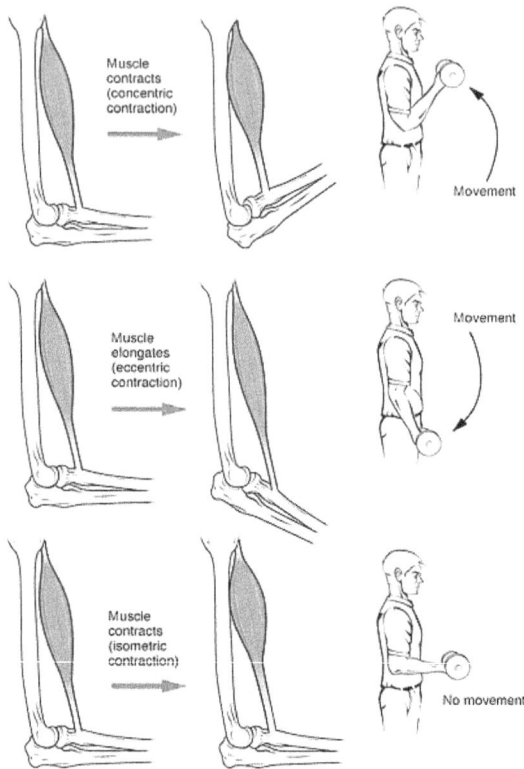

Fig. 2.20 – Examples of Eccentric and Concentric contractions
Courtesy of Creative Commons Attribution 4.0 International

Eccentric versus concentric contractions

Earlier studies among Russian weightlifters who compared their strength level when just using concentric vs. eccentric contractions showed that they were stronger when using eccentric contractions (Fig. 2.20). Recently, it has been suggested that working a muscle group in eccentric contractions using heavy weights is also more likely to cause an injury than a concentric method. Keep that in mind if you're a body builder or using heavy weights, it will vary from person to person how much is considered to be "heavy."

I'm advising here to do the last couple of reps in eccentric mode being mindful, gradual, and gentle. Posture and biomechanics will always play a significant role when using weights, or even just the weight of your own body while changing positions using the weight of gravity. Isometric exercises can help stabilize muscles and strengthen them in that position. They may help lower blood pressure if not done with intensity. (Dr. E. R. Laskowski, Mayo Clinic, 2023)

Workout tips for those who use weights and machines

Remember that anything using your arms and torso will have the potential to influence muscles in your neck (Fig. 2.21) that may also need the opportunity to unwind at the end of your workout. Saving time for a cool-down phase after these types of workouts will be well-received by your body. Engaging the triceps after doing curls will also help further release the biceps, just as engaging the rhomboids after doing bench presses will help ease the strain in the pectoralis muscles. They use the same principles of reciprocal inhibition: the antagonist releases the agonist.

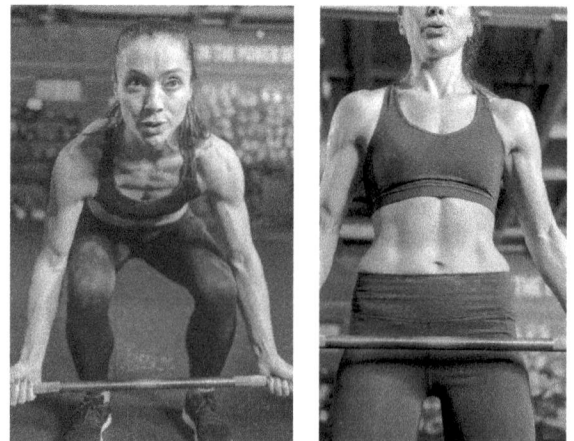

Fig. 2.21 - Example of potential strain of neck muscles and the thoracic outlet with weights

Now that we've gone over sensing through and into some of the layers that are being affected when you move, stand, sit, exercise, position yourself to sleep, or perform any activity with your body, we can begin to apply those ways of tuning in to some somatic sequences. We'll keep the midline in mind as we proceed, even as we explore finding balance using the extremities. Freedom in the midline is increased as forces that have accumulated in the arms, legs, hands, and feet are reduced. The liberated energy in the core will support the balanced use of the extremities, and vice versa.

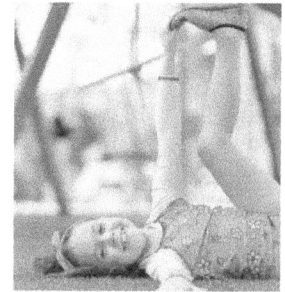

Remember the open playfulness and unbridled curiosity you had as a child or that you see children express as they play in an open field or playground. Part of what maintains their energy, is the openness and the novelty and variety of how they use their bodies, all of which feed into effortless posture. (And the fact that they're young!) Perhaps opening and releasing all the places where use patterns trap the flow of energy will be the simplest and quickest way for the body to rediscover the optimum plumb line. We'll start by finding out where you are in space already, and go from there.

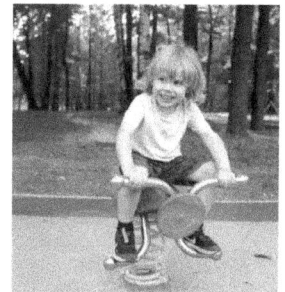

You are the fulcrum

This topic is so important in the somatic education process that I wrote an entire volume on it—Volume 7. We'll just skim over the main point in this book. Although we'll be assisting the settling of the heart using the parasympathetic plexus, the breath, and balancing the musculoskeletal, organ, and energetic systems, (and all the other things that are affected and improved by somatic principles,) what we're really needing to emphasize as a major source of input for the body is you. We've been describing various doorways into what and who you are in order to relax and settle the main point of organization: you.

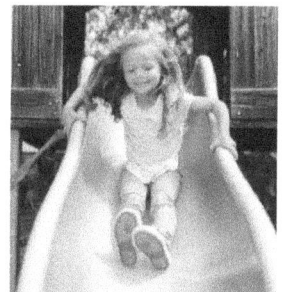

When you're settled, the heart, the breath, the muscles, and the organs will all settle more easily, and the energy and fluids will flow more freely. When you are more relaxed and more playful, more open and receptive like you were when you were a child, your system will also be more receptive, and well-being will flourish. When your mind is calmer and more meditative, your body, heart, and brain will be also. Sometimes it's easier for information to get across when it's not personal, but the fact of the matter is that your health and well-being are personal.

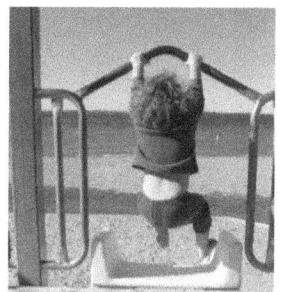

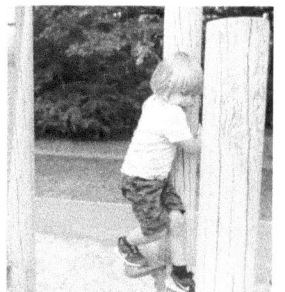

You are the point of organization; the fulcrum around which all of this works. "Alternative" methods help put you back in touch with yourself, and to become more intimate with yourself, with your body, your feelings, your senses, and how they all fit together with you and your choices. All of the above are listening for your input and pulling on past memories and associated beliefs. You are a huge part of the equation and the main prevention against auto-pilot filled with learned patterns. Typically, people want to improve their lives and health through methods that are outside of themselves—with work or entertainment, excitement, travel, being busy with social lives, or even with volunteering—all of which may be valid, fun, and useful. However, they bypass the body. The best way to reboot the body involves rest and a more specific inner focus.

Notice that the somatic methods like Feldenkrais, Hanna Somatics, Chi Kung, t'ai chi, and meditation take you through the looking glass into self-aware embodiment. Resistance may arise about processing types of approaches that involve feelings that lead to vulnerability for obvious reasons, and some people just aren't "built" that way. The feelings involved in somatic movements involve the kinesthetic "felt sense," which is different from emotions. People do vary in their capacity or propensity for sensing and will usually get into the movements without tuning in to the way it feels while doing the movements, which is fine. Part of the process involves waking up deadened cells, places where the body, and maybe even the mind have gone numb to itself.

This text will offer many ways to tune into the sensations that arise while doing the movements bcause they are a major language that the body can message you in. We'll also continue to feel into and appreciate what's under the skin while you move more into the manual therapy section of this book as well as during movement. In this case, as you open to yourself—to your inner life--and learn how to discern the responses from your body, the changes will be more immediate. In any case, it's fun and rewarding to enjoy the discoveries with your body and enjoy the new sensitivities as they develop.

Movement layers for different paths

People are organized differently for many reasons, but let's just simplify into categories of "nature versus nurture," and even preference. Most of these are learned, whether it is downloaded during embryogenesis or embodied as we take in information from family, friends, and experiences along the way. **Intellectual types** may feel more comfortable just learning to move more freely and feel less stiff at the end of the day. **Athletic types** may enjoy some specificity or proficiency in how they move after waking up receptors and connectivity throughout the system. It will enhance performance, flexibility, and fluidity.

Dancers and other **performing arts professionals** may appreciate the sensory exploration more because it deepens their ability to connect with themselves and how they express through their bodies. **Emotional types** may be open to examining where mental and emotional tensions are held and enjoy the process and sensation of them being discharged. **Inward, sensitive types** like meditators, therapists, and moving arts enthusiasts may embrace the nuances of the energy, blissful sensitivity, and spaciousness that becomes more available when tuning into the finer discriminations in the wakefulness of the tissues. These are, of course, only generalizations that don't always apply according to these categorizations.

Of course, these traits may appear in a myriad of combinations, so don't feel pigeon-holed in any way. It's possible for a person to fit all categories. There are also different learning styles within the categories of personality types and activity leanings. What you enjoy or are pulled to during the process over time may change; different doors of perception may open and lead to new, exciting, rewarding discoveries and benefits. It's all good. As we proceed into the movements themselves, three layers of specificity will be included. You can choose, for any or all movement sequences, which level you'd like to explore or what you feel you have time for on any given day.

The somatic groups will be as follows:

- ➲ Simple description of the movement for the three categories (Group 1)
- ➲ Movement description, plus sensation tracking with breath (Group 2)
- ➲ The above plus listening and waiting for feedback from the body before the next move (Group 3)

For everyone it always elevates the experience when you find the pleasure and enjoyment of being in touch with your body as it moves.

> 99 _____
>
> *Outside of the physical, Mind is ever active and able to alter the physical as well as the non-physical. The healing of the psyche occurs simultaneously if we realize the inseparability of mental/emotional, and physical attributes.*
>
> *R. Paul Lee, D.O.*
>
> _____ 99

CHAPTER 3
Clearing the Path of the Heart

We've discussed the studies that revealed why the heart is so vulnerable, covered the aspects of life that have the most impact before and after birth, and mentioned some preventative measures to help maintain its health over time. A great deal of what ages the heart, besides air quality, is mental and emotional status. Candace Pert pioneered groundbreaking research in the 1980s that discovered that specific peptides acted as biochemical messengers that had target receptors in numerous areas of the body, including organs, glands, nerve cells, intestines, and the immune system. It was also discovered that certain types of thoughts could trigger emotions that would light up particular pathways where these peptides had been traced with dye.

The body is a mirror

Author Pilar Gerasimo describes the phenomena like this: "It turns out that biochemical reactions to mental and emotional stimuli – your everyday thoughts and feelings – occur not just in the brain, but also, often simultaneously, in virtually every system of your body." Part of how **neuropeptides** function is as an interpreter of cues in the environment in relation to the needs of the person for food, safety, sleep, mating, movement, and basic survival mechanisms. As such, they are wired into the central nervous system (CNS) for fight and flight and can become vulnerable to mixed messages that lead to anxiety, depression, addictions, sleep disorders, and more. Gerasimo goes on to say:

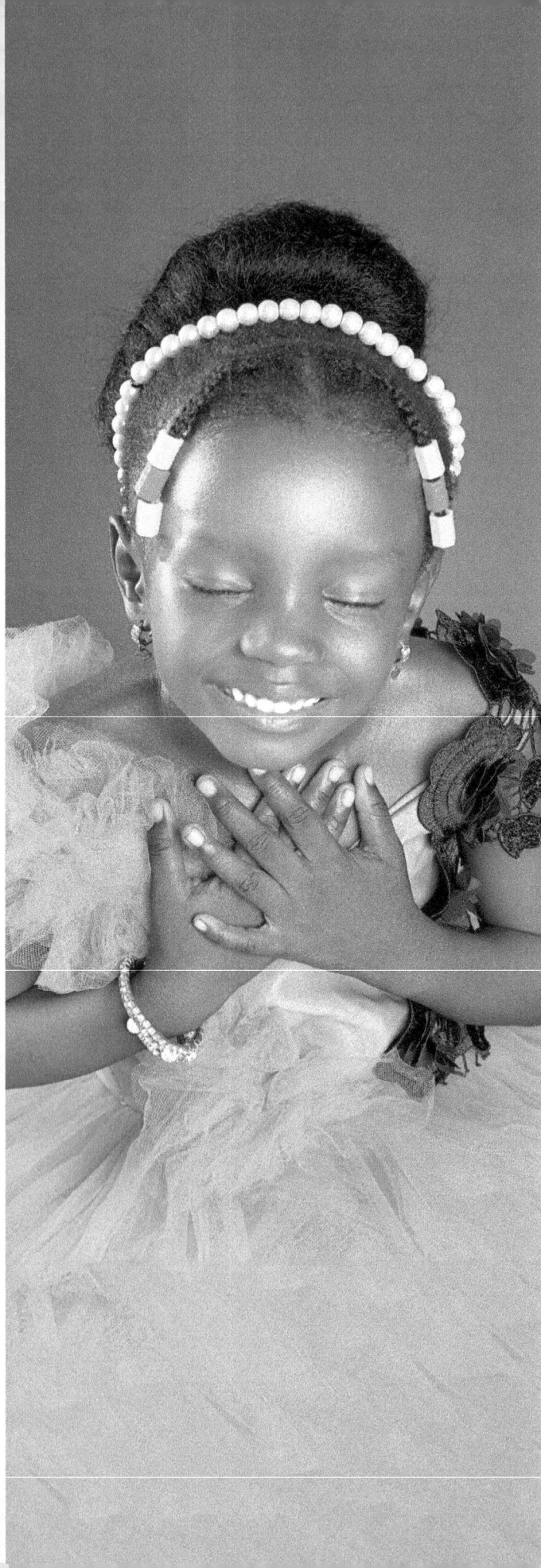

> *If you even remotely grasp the roles played by peptides, cell-receptors and synapses in creating your biochemical profile, and you understand generally how emotion both catalyzes and is catalyzed by them, then you are part of a small but growing group of people getting in on the front end of one of the most interesting stories to hit health and wellness circles this century. Unfortunately, it is also one of the most underreported stories in recent memory.* (Pilar Gerasimo, *"Emotional Biochemistry"*, Experience Life, Brain Health/Functional/Integrative Medicine, November 2020)[40]

Pert's discovery of the opiate receptor during her doctorate work at Johns Hopkins University in the 1970s led to her being a recipient of the coveted Lasker Award, also known as the "American Nobel Prize." It also led to the field of psychoneuroimmunology, as it proved the connection between thoughts, emotions, and health by way of their influence on biological systems. She calls the body our "subconscious mind," and stated, **Mind doesn't dominate body, it becomes body.** Shaman who have grown up with this understanding know how to transmute and release blocked emotions using psychoactive substances in rituals designed in a reverent way. Westerners have often sought out these practices or have attempted to target those receptors in other ways.

Neuropeptide receptors are found in many places along emotional circuits. They are cues to approach, avoid, and motivating behaviors related to survival such as anger, fear, sadness, disgust, happiness, and a host of both pleasant and unpleasant emotions. (Nummenmaa and Touminen, *"Opioid system and human emotions,"* British Journal of Pharmacology, 175(14), 2017)[41] There is a reward system in the brain that is independent of dopamine. It could be that the brain rewards movement because it means that you may be moving toward food or social interaction that could help provide food, protection, or mating—all related to survival. But I believe that there's a higher order of reward that happens because it's rewarding to connect with yourself.

Movement also has contact with opiate receptors and can trigger **endorphins**. That's why they call it a 'runner's high' and why some people get **addicted**. I've heard many stories from patients with bone-on-bone scenarios in their knees or hips who refused to stop running. It seems to take moderately intense or extended exercise to trigger the release of those endorphins, which can also at times act as an endogenous analgesic, or pain reliever. In fact, research shows that some types of vigorous exercise ease aches and pains. (Paul Govern, *"Study finds aerobic exercise spurs endorphins, relieves low back pain,"* Vanderbilt University Medical Center Reporter, August 5, 2020) [42]

While there are many benefits to exercising at these levels, there are other ways to trigger 'feel good' chemicals in the body outside of the 'no pain, no gain' point of view. The body most likely realizes that it's also beneficial and healthy to be present and aware in your body without intensity or intense arousal. In fact, many ailments self-correct during slow, gentle movements.

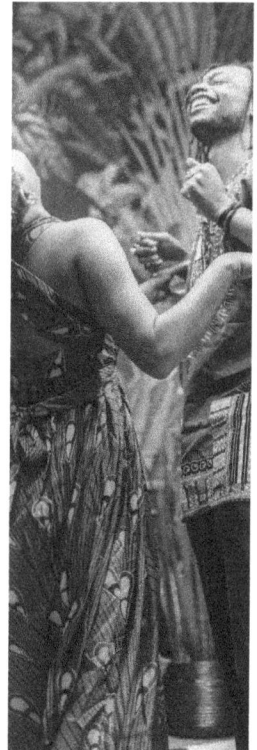

How movement improves almost everything

The ancient traditions of yoga and qi gong help foster integrated balance and harmony in the body and mind. (Paula Boaventura, et al., *"Yoga and Qigong for Health: Two Sides of the Same Coin?"* Behavioral Sciences, 2022 July 12(7):222)[43] After reviewing 145 studies comparing the benefits of these movement practices, Boaventura and her team reported:

Yoga

- ⮕ Significant reduction in C-reactive protein (inflammatory marker) and other .....inflammatory responses in chronic disease for some participants
- ⮕ Reduction in back pain
- ⮕ Lowered psychological distress
- ⮕ Increased energy levels

Qi Gong

- ⮕ Significantly reduced pain intensity
- ⮕ Improved functional issues in the spine
- ⮕ Decreased heart and respiratory rates
- ⮕ Increased core muscle strength and range of motion
- ⮕ Improved mental status

(All in comparison to office workers in the study who didn't participate in the activity)

There are several other studies that may need larger samples to be definitive, but are seeing benefits in blood pressure, blood sugar, sleep disorders, PTSD, mood and anxiety disorders, mild cognitive impairment, and various menopausal symptoms in either qi gong or yoga. Both have positive effects on the parasympathetic response, and yoga in particular has been shown to be neuroprotective and generate larger brain volume in areas involved in body representation, attention, self-relevant processing, visualization, and stress regulation. It also stimulates a vagal response which can improve overall functioning of many systems. The researchers caution that other forms of exercise that have not been as widely studied may provide similar benefits, such as **Feldenkrais** and **Hanna Somatic Education**. There are numerous reports of pain relief, restored mobility, a sense of increased balance and connectedness, and deep relaxation using these modalities. They also provides classes nationwide, some of which are online.

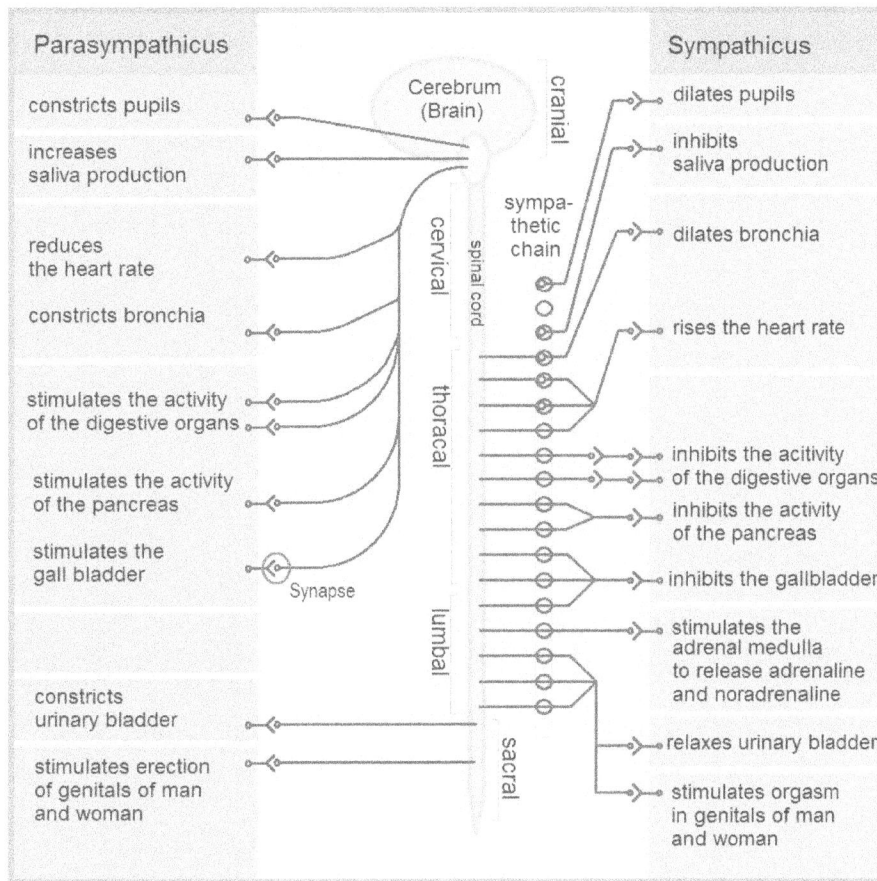

Fig. 3.1 – Function of the Autonomic Nervous System *(potentially influenced by movement)*
Courtesy of Medium69, JMarchn, CC BY-SA 4.0 via Wikimedia Commons

Movement is medicine

The main takeaway from these studies and personal experience, is that movement is indeed medicine (Fig. 3.1). The process of opening the flow of chi or prana, which is nourishing to the system and supports neurophysiological balance, reduces tightness and tension as it feeds tissue fields, stimulates proprioceptors in joints and connective tissue, while moving fluids and breath. Improving the flow through the midline can directly improve overall functioning. Yoga and qi gong can be considered to be forms of moving meditation, as can many forms of Hanna Somatics or Feldenkrais. Perhaps pilates and other forms of movement-based practices in which conscious attention and self-regulation are required can be thought of in the same way. There is a certain amount of self-regulatory activity that becomes stimulated during any form of exercise as it wakes the body up into a cascade of biochemical responses that can be very helpful if not healing.

Movement is bliss

Endorphins and dopamine are not the only source of euphoria generated by exercise. The body also produces **endocannabinoids**, such as anandamide and something called 2- AG, or 2-arachidonoglycerol. 2-AG plays an essential role in balancing pain sensation, inflammation, synaptic plasticity, the stress response, cognition, emotion, and energy balance. (Hemraj and Jassey, 2023) [44] They both bind to CB1 and CB2 receptors all over the rest of the body (Fig. 3.2) and seem to act as **neuromodulators**.

Endocannabinoids are known to help pain and inflammation, but they also help spasticity in epilepsy and multiple sclerosis, and appetite stimulation for cancer patients. (Pertwee and Ross, 2002; Dietrich and McDaniel, 2004)[45] They don't have psychotropic effects. Due to the abundance of CB1 receptors in the brain, particularly in the hippocampus, brain stem, neocortex, basal ganglia, and cerebellum, they are being studied for their potential benefits in neurodegenerative conditions.

CANNABINOID RECEPTORS IN THE BODY

CB1

CB2

CB1

PERIPHERAL/CENTRAL NERVOUS SYSTEM
BRAIN AND SPINAL CORD
PITUITARY, THYROID, ADRENAL GLANDS
DIGESTIVE TRACT
MUSCLE CELLS
LIVER CELLS
FAT CELLS
PLACENTA
OVARIES
KIDNEYS
RETINA
LUNGS
SPERM

CB2

PERIPHERAL NERVOUS SYSTEM AND BRAIN
REPRODUCTIVE SYSTEM
DIGESTIVE TRACT
ADIPOSE TISSUE
THYMUS
BONE MARROW
IMMUNE CELLS
KIDNEYS AND LIVER
PANCREAS
TONSILS
SPLEEN
SKIN
EYE

Fig. 3.2 – Illustration of the where the endogenous cannabinoids, anandamide and 2-AG, bind to CB1 and CB2 receptors in the body.
Courtesy of Creative Commons Attribution 4.0 International

Called the '**bliss molecule**' by some researchers, **anandamide** doesn't require a great deal of exercise intensity to be released. (Michael Siebers, et al., *"Exercise-induced euphoria and anxiolysis (sedation) do not depend on endogenous opioids in humans,"* Psychoneuroendocrinology, Vol. 126, April 2021)[46] Exercise is being used as a substitution therapy for opioid addiction, as it has shown multiple benefits both physically and mentally including the reduction of substance use. (Alexandros Serianos, et al., *The Role of Physical Exercise in Opioid Substitution Therapy: Mechanisms of Sequential Effects*, IJMS, 21 February 2023)[47] The bottom line is that the body lets you know in multiple ways, that movement is rewarding, and these are the mechanisms whereby the system can let you know you did a good thing. There are also types of bliss that are just inherent in what we are (kundalini and anandamaya kosha-the bliss body), that can be awakened and accessed. They are not dependent upon movement and answer to Divine Grace.

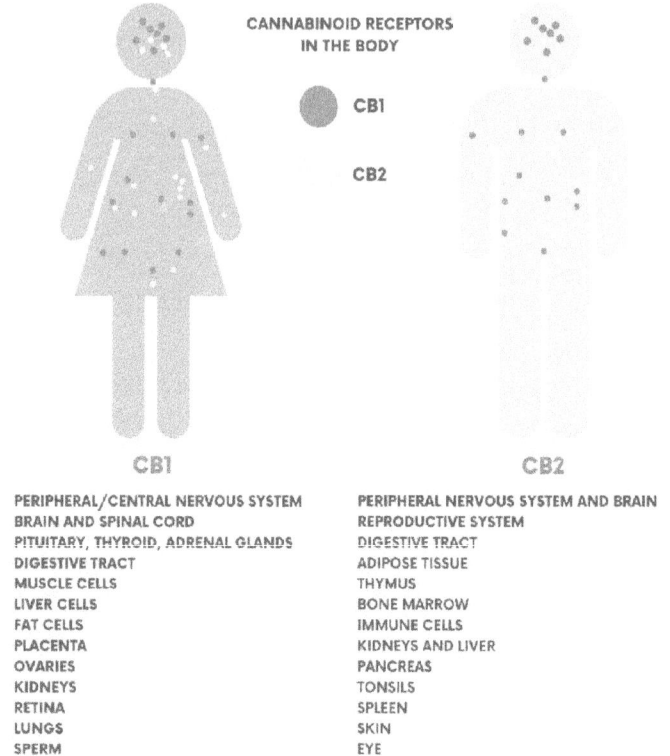

Getting in touch

You can produce the same rewards for yourself by using manual therapy methods to release tightness and tension while increasing the flow of energy, fluids and breath. You will still be present and listening to your body while manually opening many tissue layers, fluid flow, and joints. In either case, you will be both increasing awareness and awakening the cells and their varied functions. In the process you'll be part of the feedback and feedforward loops that inform you and your body how things are going as it literally shifts under your touch. Recall the ways in which you touch something or someone you care about and how it feels when someone you care about touches you. Consider bringing that same care and sensitivity into play when you make contact with yourself.

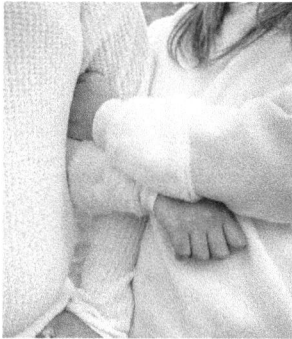

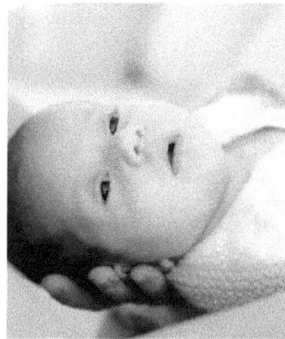

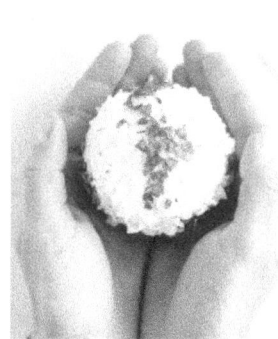

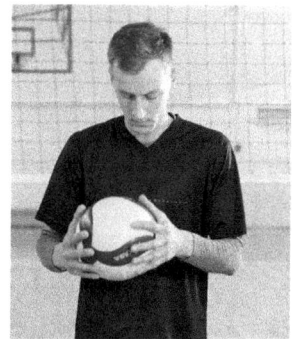

Explore the difference you might experience if you move as though you love **what** you're moving, and you love **that** you're moving—like it's your favorite time in your day and you can't wait to get into every part of it. Pause before beginning the movement or the manual therapy methods we'll learn, and bring as much care and sensitivity to it as you would if you were sharing it with a dear, close friend. It bears repeating that the cells are listening to your every thought and feeling, and they are responding in kind. The cells will mirror the way you are truly thinking and feeling, as they are one with those parts of you, and respond biochemically based on those cues. In the same way, joyful movement is transduced into biochemical messengers that are epigenetic and transformative. This approach stimulates the release of "bliss" molecules if not oxytocin into your system.

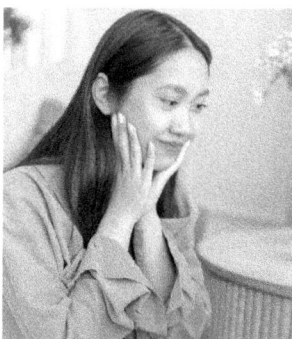

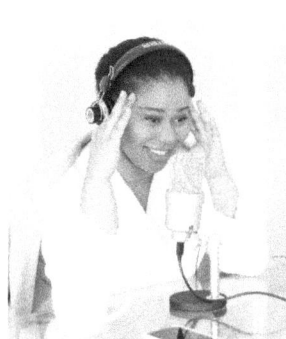

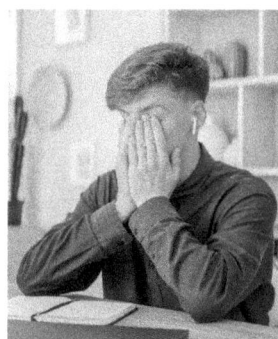

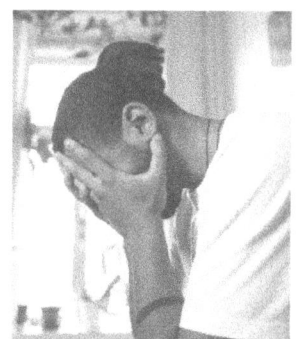

ONE SKY

Consider the many times and ways that you naturally touch your face in times of overwork or overwhelm, when you intuitively know how to comfort yourself. In this case, you will just explore how it feels to make the contact more conscious and intentional, in a way that communicates safety and caring to your body. These movement sequences and manual therapy sequences will benefit from you treating them as a place and time to comfort and nourish yourself. For Group #1 who will just be moving, you can just move and ignore the touchy-feely part.

Starting from neutral

There are many pages in Volume 7 on posture, but let's go over it briefly here in the interest of the plumb line, the midline, and starting from a neutral place in the system. There is a greater probability that your body will be attentive to new movements that change old patterns if it begins with minimum strain. Having a more open, balanced midline will also provide more energy and conductivity through which the information can transmit the movement options, and you will be able to more easily sense the feedback your body provides.

Use a mirror initially so you can check where your body is currently in relation the plumb line and bony landmarks in the center of gravity. Facing front, check the bony landmarks at the front of your pelvis for an anterior rotation or a counter-rotation (as mentioned in the last chapter (2.13 and 2.14). Place your fingers horizontally on each ASIS (green arrows) and notice if your fingers are at the same level or not (Fig.3.3).

If the right ASIS is low, as can often happen while driving, then you could do a lunge with the left leg back to help even it out. (Fig. 3.4)

If there is a counter-rotation with the left ilium behind the right one, then during the lunge, swivel the left hip in your stance until it's slightly in front of the right one, then recheck when you finish the lunge.

If the left ASIS is behind the right one when you look down at your fingers, then there is a counter-rotation from leading with the right leg while sitting, hiking, biking, surfing, etc.

Remind yourself to lead with the left leg from time to time— pulling with the left (quads) and pushing with the right side (hamstrings). If in a chair, let your knees be even, even if your feet are not.

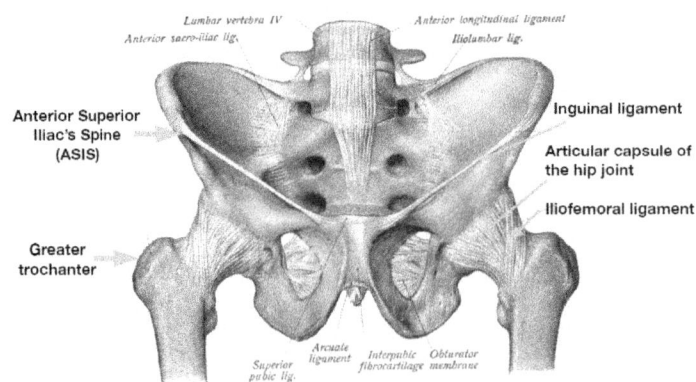

Labels on figure:
Lumbar vertebra IV
Anterior sacro-iliac lig.
Anterior longitudinal ligament
Iliolumbar lig.
Anterior Superior Iliac's Spine (ASIS)
Inguinal ligament
Articular capsule of the hip joint
Iliofemoral ligament
Greater trochanter
Arcuate ligament
Superior pubic lig.
Interpubic fibrocartilage
Obturator membrane

Fig. 3.3 - *Landmarks of the pelvis*

Using the runners' lunge to correct the ASIS (anterior rotation)

While in the lunge position, have your arms up and notice whether there are areas in the shoulder girdle or in the abdominal cavity - medial or lateral, upper or lower sections – that feel a little more resistant to lengthening than other areas. If there are:

- Pull your shoulder blades down toward your waist as you arch your back slightly, then flatten your back as you lift again. Repeat twice.

- Inhale, exhale, and pull one blade down as you side-bend slightly to that side, and repeat on the other side.

- Inhale, exhale and lean forward and down toward your navel with your ribs. Then come up, breathe and drop the ribs on the right, come up, breathe and repeat on the left.

- Recheck and notice if it feels more balanced for your shoulders and abdomen while in the lunge position.

- Now go back to the mirror and see if you've been able to adjust the pelvic alignment into a more balanced place. Be aware that if you've had a C-section or abdominal surgery, there may be changes to this area leading to more resistance or stiffness in the area of the scar tissue.

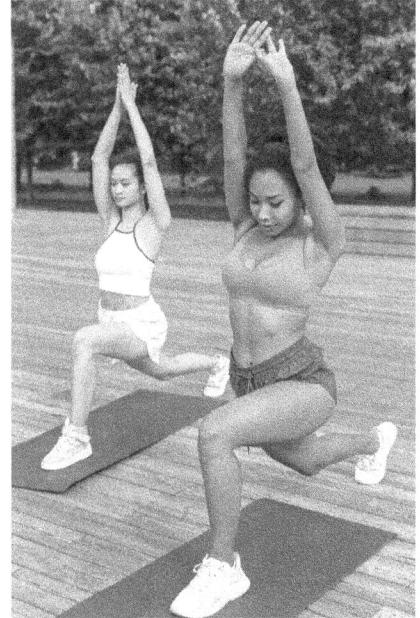

Fig. 3.4 – Runners' Lunge with arms up to help release the muscles in the abdominal cavity that might contribute to the shift in pelvic balance.

Finding neutral posture

When the center of gravity is balanced, we can sense neutral posture and find the plumb line more easily. First, notice where you are on your feet. Lean forward and back until you feel that your weight is just below your ankles: behind the balls of your feet but in front of your heels. Notice whether you feel your quads being engaged, your hamstrings, or, optimally, neither. This means you're really standing in and through your bones with your weight-bearing. This is how you find it whenever you want to. You're balanced front to back, now balance side-to-side. Lean over to the right side and then gradually over to the left, until you feel your weight in the middle of the feet, and are not engaging the iliotibial tract or the adductors (Fig. 3.5).

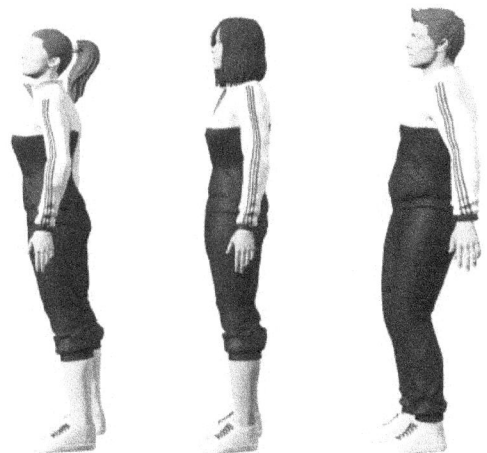

Test yourself by swaying gently and slowly in and back out of each direction. Notice which position you're in when a particular muscle group is activated. Check to see where the balanced position creates the most ease in your knees and ankles. You want to try and let the skeleton do as much of the work as possible without the muscles in your legs engaging any more than necessary.

One of the reasons it's so important to start in a neutral posture is that it's possible to compound the strains and imbalances in your body if you don't find a neutral baseline and learn how to sense where that is and when it feels off. Sensing where it's off means you can also learn how to correct it by sensation alone. Look in the mirror if you need to, but your body will produce discomfort if the compensatory patterns are corrected and the cells have been awakened. When the muscles are imbalanced, all types of distortions can happen in the skeleton (Fig. 3.6). Even mild to moderate changes will still be significant and potentially set up the system for back pain, hip dysfunction, and knee problems.

In this case, the thorax and pelvis are rotated right, while the legs and feet are still pointed straight. The left ilium is elevated, or it could be the classic anterior rotation of the right ilium. The left ilium shows an inflare with a shortened space between the ribs and pelvis on the left side, with the beginning of a slight scoliosis on that side. The head is rotated opposite the pelvis, likely to counter-balance.

We can assume which muscle groups are responsible for this skeletal rearrangement, but the main point to realize is that when the muscles shift, the bones do as well; when the position in gravity shifts, the muscles will also be offset. As we move into the next section of self-sensing that is also self-correcting as you go, pay attention to differences in sensation that may be produced by muscles being tighter on one side than another.

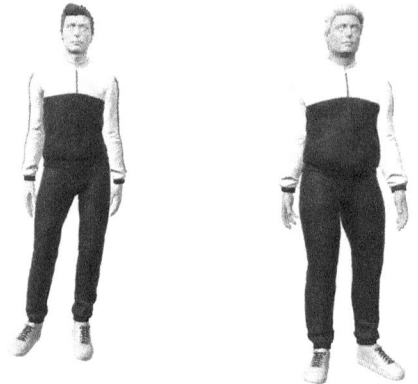

Fig. 3.5 - Lean to the left and to the right, feeling where the tension lands in your legs and feet until you find the most neutral place.

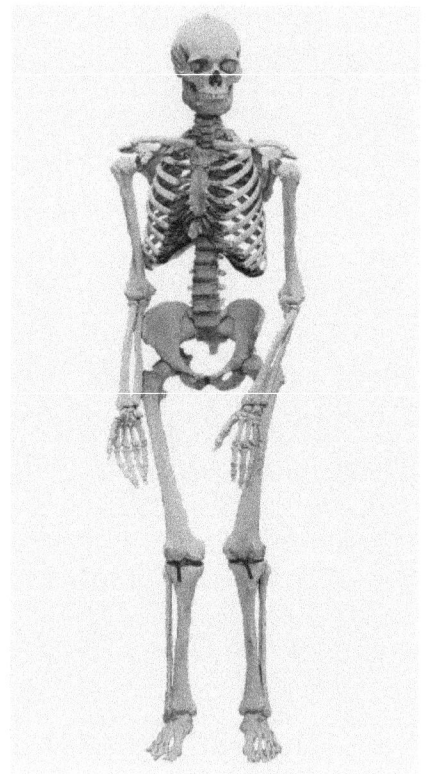

Fig. 3.6 – Postural distortions influence right down to the bone, causing further muscular imbalances
Courtesy of Creative Commons Attribution 4.0, International

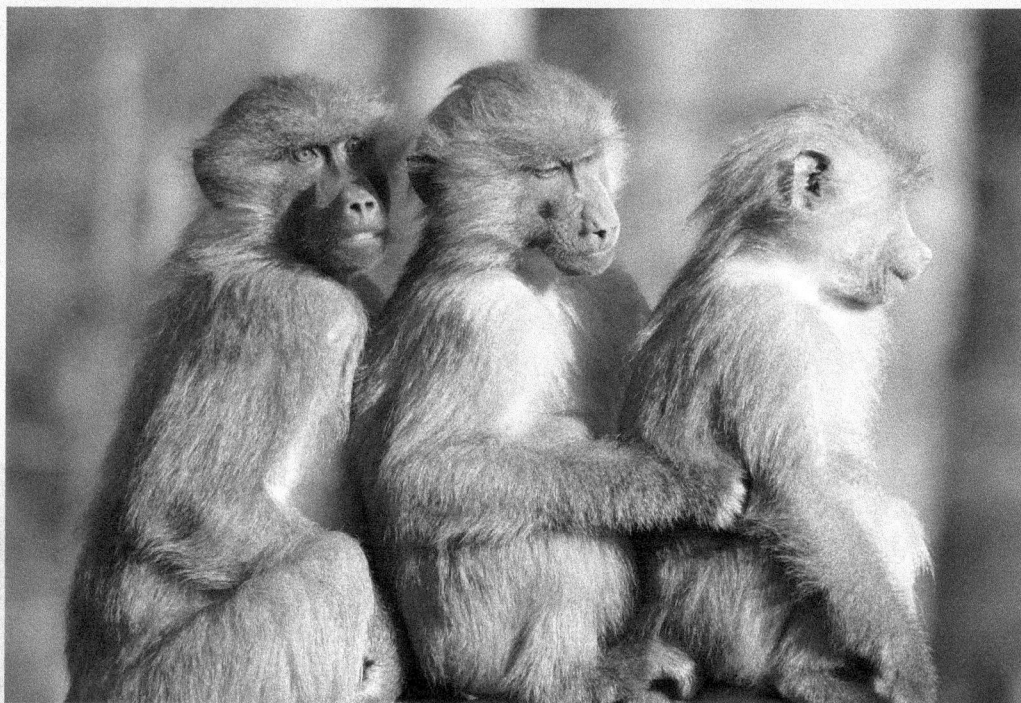

Section 2

Manual Therapy for the Midline While Standing

Easy self-adjustments you can make to ease tension and to regain or retain balance, calmness, and centeredness

> **"** _____
>
> *The fascia is not only the dwelling place of the soul (life), but also where the seeds of disease germinate. A knowledge of the universal extent of the fascia is imperative, and is one one of the greatest aids to the person who seeks the causes of disease.*
>
>
>
> *A. T. Still*
>
> _____ **"**
>
>

Myofascial Arch and Curl

Start low and walk both hands upward ^ Stretch the skin up as you go ^ Arch and curl as your hands walk up

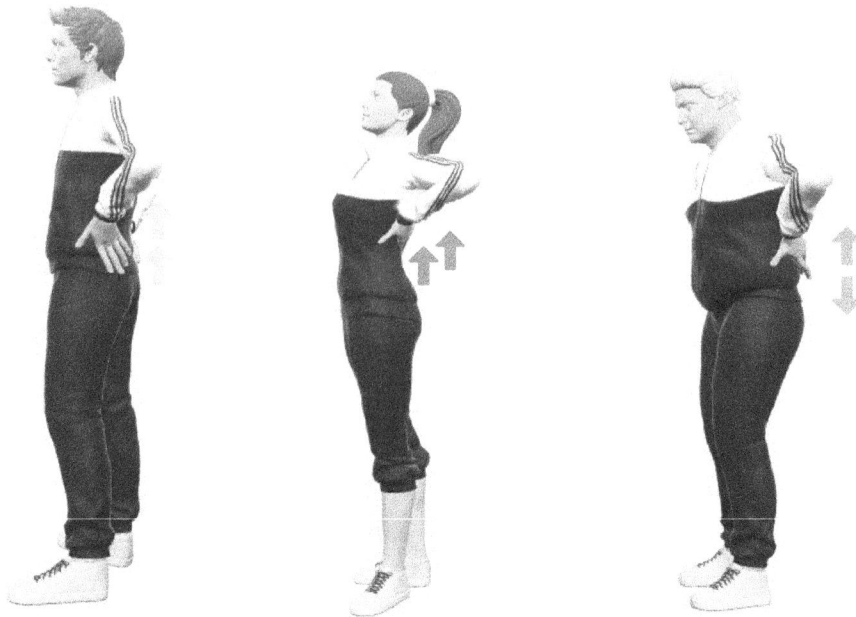

Exploring the ease of midline extension and flexion while standing

Group 1: Movement description

After finding balanced posture on your feet, place your hands on your hips alongside your sacrum and gently arch, then slowly curl your back (tuck your butt under in flexion). If any place feels sore or achy, stop and go the opposite direction and come back to it even more slowly.

Don't push through it; wait for it to yield. Repeat the arch and curl 3 times with your hands in this first position before moving them up the back an inch. Lift/stretch the skin upward slightly as you do the movement.

Repeat the flexion and extension of the spine and sacrum 2 to 3 times with each hand position. Only go as far in any direction with the arching and curling as you know is comfortable. It's okay to move through stiffness, but not pain. Come back to any stiff areas and repeat the arch and curl to see if they've improved and feel freer.

Group 2: Track sensations as you move and breathe

Take a deep breath into your belly, and stretch the skin up slightly where your hands are on your sacrum. Exhale slowly as you arch, flatten and tuck your low back and sacrum. Notice where it may feel a little tighter as you move, and move more slowly in those areas.

Repeat the movements 3 times before walking your hands up an inch to the next higher spot alongside your spine. Do you notice any changes in the sacrum as your hand position changes? Is there any pull down the back of the legs? Does it feel easier with each repetition?

Do any segments or vertebrae feel a little pinchy when you arch? Is the sensation on the right, on the left, or in the middle? Place your fingers closer to that spot and inhale, hold it for 3 seconds, then exhale and continue up the spine. Return to the bottom, walk up again with just one breath at each level, and compare to how it felt the first time through the sequence.

Group 3: Move, sense, breathe, and listen and allow

As you place your hands on your sacrum, adjust them according to the location that produces the most relaxation in your hips and back. Take a deep belly breath, pause for your system to reorganize, and pause again as you stretch the skin upwards, giving your system a few seconds to shift again. It typically will relax more after each input.

Notice which level in the spine and which side of the spine responds more quickly or doesn't seem to let go. Pause at that segment and hold the in breath for 3 seconds to see whether that segment prefers an arch or a cur, then exhale and hold the out breath for 3 seconds. Did it let go more?

Do the same for the flattening and tucking under of the low back and sacrum, noticing whether this position or the exhale is preferred for the sluggish area of the spine or sacrum. Sense whether the resistance is coming from the transverse or spinous processes (Fig. 3.7), the disc in between, or the muscles adjacent to the vertebrae?

Find a spot in another area of the spine that has a similar sensation and pair them, with one hand on the lower spot, and one hand on the higher one. Inhale, hold, wait for the body to acknowledge and respond (soften, open, lengthen), then exhale and do the same. If no other spot feels similar, then straddle that vertebrae with your fingers and apply the aforementioned. This works well for scoliosis.

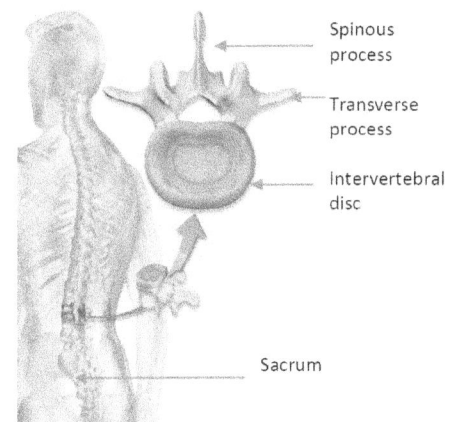

Fig. 3.7 – Spine with vertebral segment illustrated
Courtesy of BruceBlaus, CC BY-SA 4.0 via Wikimedia Commons

The muscles on the "high rib" side of an idiopathic scoliosis (onset at puberty) will be very different from the other side (Fig.3.8). Although these types of presentations can change in a way that straightens the spine, the ribs will remain in their altered position. A great deal of softening and increased relaxation can happen, so if by chance you have scoliosis that is mild or moderate, these movements will still have benefit.

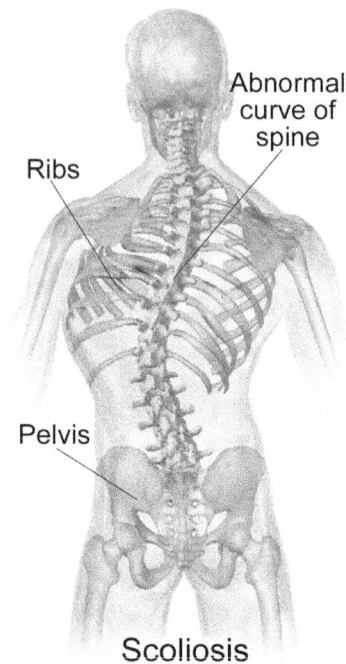

Abnormal curve of spine

Ribs

Pelvis

Scoliosis

Fig. 3.8-Idiopathic scoliosis
Courtesy of Creative Commons Attribution 3.0 Unported

It is also very possible that posture is impacted by internal organ position, function, and freedom. The issues can begin in the viscera or organs. Remember that there are layers of soft tissue, fascia, adhesions, and other membranes such as the parietal peritoneum mentioned earlier that can restrict motion of the thorax (Fig.2.11) and affect the spine.

Chronic stress can impact the vagus nerve that runs along the midline and can also have an effect on the internal organs and how well they're functioning. It has been tagged the 'wandering nerve' because after it leaves the brain stem as a cranial nerve, it wanders down through the neck and throat, chest, and abdomen, influencing practically everything of significance along the way (Fig. 3.9).

One reason the vagus nerve has become so popular recently is that so many health issues stem from it being compressed, inflamed, or irritated in some way, even by virtue of stress or infection. Some common issues it has been associated with include irregular heartbeat, indigestion, or even Crohn's disease, heartburn and bloating, chronic pain, fatigue, tinnitus, headaches, anxiety, and dizziness.

When we address structures along the midline, we will be having an influence on the vagus nerve. We may not feel the nerve itself but may instead notice a resolution of symptoms. Later in the text we'll be contacting the focal points of the parasympathetic plexuses at the cranial base and sacrum.

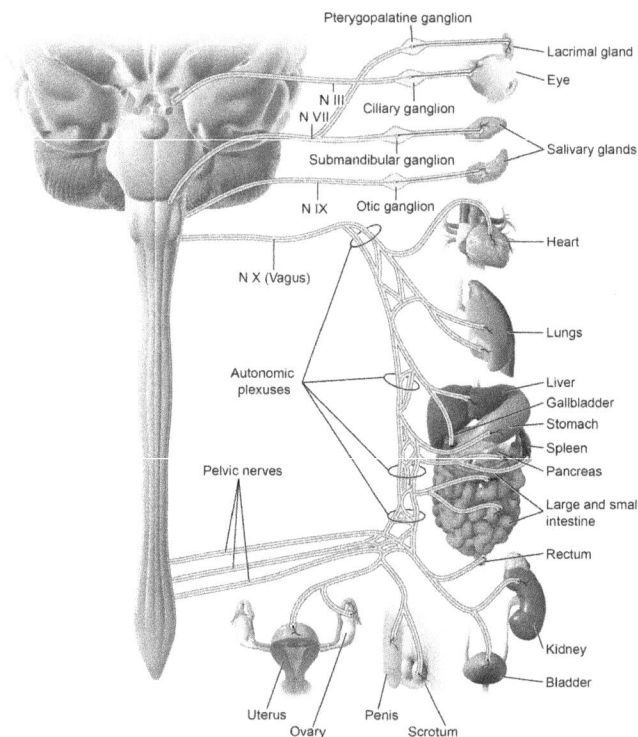

Fig. 3.9 – Parasympathetic Nervous system and its connections to the embryological endoderm layer: the senses and associated cranial nerves, internal organs, viscera, and urogenital organs.
(Image courtesy of Blausen.com staff (2014). "Medical gallery of Blausen Medical 2014." WikiJournal of Medicine 1(2)DOI:10. 15347/w/m/2014 010. ISSN 2002-4436, CC BY-SA 3.0 via Wikimedia Commons

Pairing related midline structures while standing

There are many times when the location of tension is not the source of it. We've been exploring the relationships between a variety of structures based on the fact that they are in constant communication with one another. Now that postural corrections have enhanced their ability to signal each other and have a more efficient response, let's put some of the major nerve plexus, organs, glands, and energy centers in intentional contact. Because the parasympathetic nervous system, the cardiovascular system, digestive and immune systems, lymphatic system, viscera, and major meridians will be addressed, the result will be immediately soothing, calming, releasing, and relaxing on many levels.

Parasympathetic Manual Therapy Sequence 1

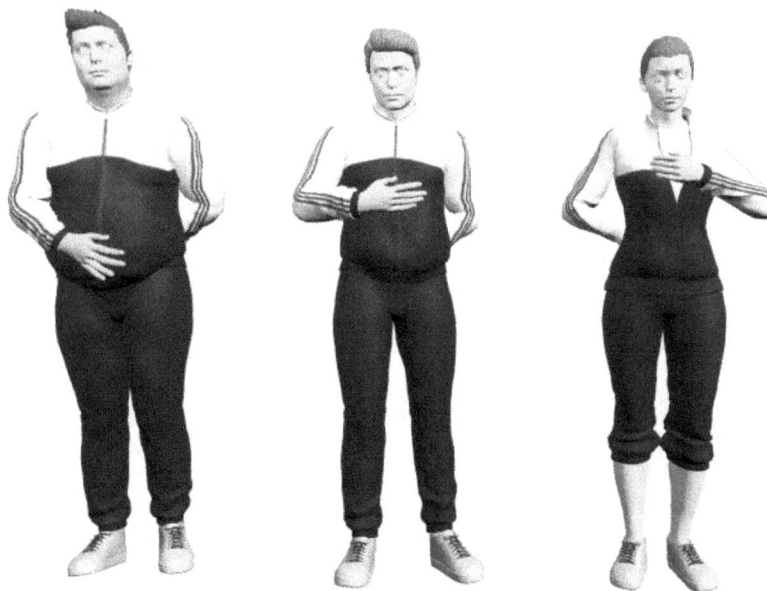

A-Sacrum and the belly   B-Sacrum and the solar plexus   C-Sacrum and the heart

Start by leaving one hand comfortably on your sacrum. This place is just opposite the center of gravity—an energy storage place in chi kung called the dan tian, which means 'field of elixir.' It is also contacting part of the parasympathetic plexus at S2 and S3, which has an effect on urogenital and bowel function. There are numerous stabilizing ligaments that criss-cross over the sacrum, along with several muscle attachments from the back and hip muscles. In short, it is a powerful place for you to hold and pair with other significant structures of the midline. It is also above the second chakra, which, according to some theories, governs emotions, sexuality, vitality, and creativity. These hand positions also have the potential of benefiting all of the organs in your body.

Group 1: Be present with a gentle touch

Close your eyes and have your thumb over your belly button while the rest of your hand rests over your intestines (A). Count to 10, then move that hand up to your solar plexus (B). After 10 seconds, move the hand up to your heart (C), and count to 10 again.

Group 2: Sense and breathe

Take deep breath into your belly as you place your hand there, and be aware of the changes that may happen in the abdominal cavity, lower back, legs, and feet. After 10 seconds, exhale and move that hand up to your solar plexus.

Inhale and notice if the adjacent organs produce any sensations or adjust their position while your hand is there. Notice the sound or sensation of arteries reflecting the heartbeat.

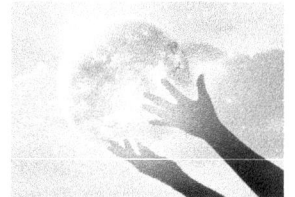

Exhale after 10 seconds, then inhale again as you move your hand up to the area of your heart. Close your eyes and be aware of sensations that may arise throughout your system. Exhale. Repeat while imagining a golden ball of light at each contact point.

Group 3: Sense, breathe, pause, and listen

Following the timing and breath suggestions from the previous group, pause as soon as you make contact and notice how and where your body responds. Wait for it to complete its motion and modifications before moving your hands to the next station. Change the amount of pressure slightly on your sacrum and notice if there is more release in the hips afterwards.

Check to see which hand positions are the most impactful for you; which ones have the most global effect. If your body moves into a position that's out of midline, pause and wait for it to complete its process there, after which it will return to midline. Test whether the inbreath or the out breath is the most supportive for its return to midline. Return to the hand combination that has the most global effect, and take a few breaths there to finish the sequence.

These movement and sensing explorations with the hand on the sacrum have the potential to also have a positive influence on several muscle groups in the back (Fig.3.9) and legs (Fig.3.10), including the intricate, intrinsic ones that are right next to the spine, in between the transverse and spinous processes. Releasing them can be a big help in relieving stiffness and improving flexibility.

Remember that all of the nerve roots that innervate the hips and legs exit the spine and sacrum where you'll be touching. In addition, the nerve bundles exiting the spinal cord (Cauda equine and filum terminale) will be under your hands at the sacrum, having the potential to release muscles higher up as well.

What you're touching and influencing

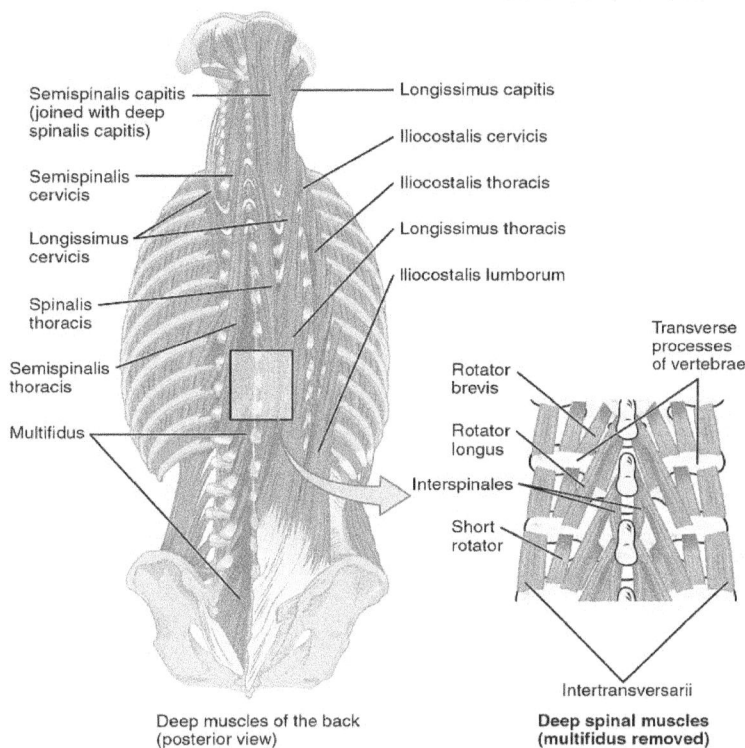

Semispinalis capitis
(joined with deep
spinalis capitis)

Semispinalis
cervicis

Longissimus
cervicis

Spinalis
thoracis

Semispinalis
thoracis

Multifidus

Longissimus capitis

Iliocostalis cervicis

Iliocostalis thoracis

Longissimus thoracis

Iliocostalis lumborum

Transverse
processes
of vertebrae

Rotator
brevis

Rotator
longus

Interspinales

Short
rotator

Intertransversarii

Deep muscles of the back
(posterior view)

**Deep spinal muscles
(multifidus removed)**

Fig. 3.9 – Illustration of paravertebral muscles in detail
Image courtesy of OpenStax 4.0 via Wikimedia commons

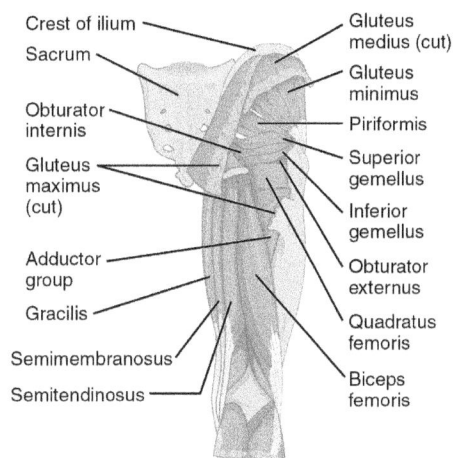

Crest of ilium

Sacrum

Obturator
internis

Gluteus
maximus
(cut)

Adductor
group

Gracilis

Semimembranosus

Semitendinosus

Gluteus
medius (cut)

Gluteus
minimus

Piriformis

Superior
gemellus

Inferior
gemellus

Obturator
externus

Quadratus
femoris

Biceps
femoris

Fig. 3.10 – Muscles of the hip that attach to the sacrum and move the leg.
Courtesy of OpenStax College, CC BY 3.0 via Wikimedia Commons

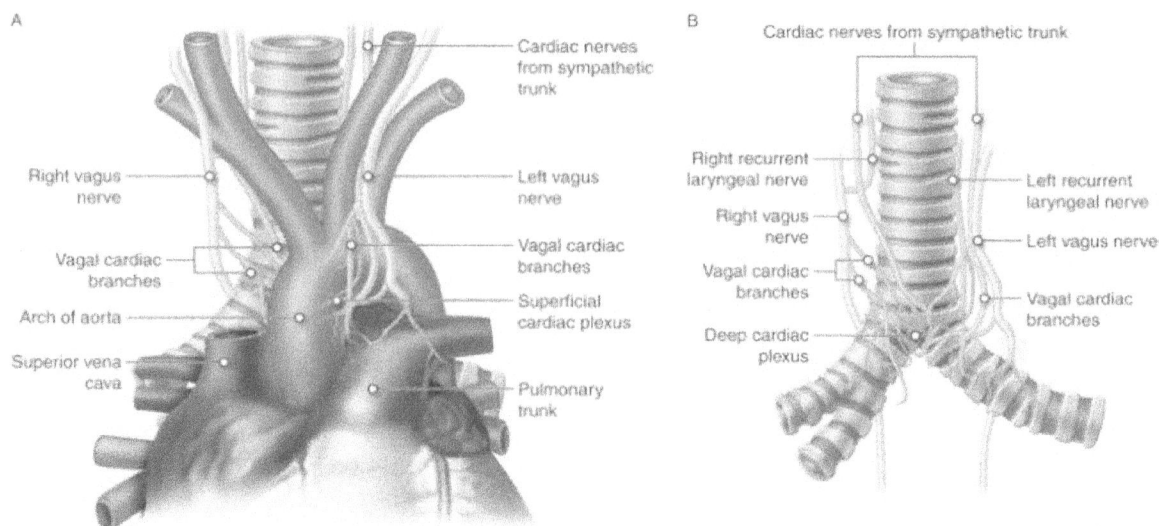

Fig. 3.11 – Cardiac plexus and vagus nerve
Courtesy of Cenveo, CC BY 4.0, via Wikimedia Commons

There are both sympathetic and parasympathetic nerve fibers in and around the heart (Fig.3.11). We began this book speaking about the importance of heart health and the fact that it, along with the intestines, is imbedded with tens of thousands of nerve cells, making them both qualify as a brain. Creating a state of harmony and coherence within and between each of these systems can make a big difference in stress reduction as well as in overall well-being. These simple explorations can supply great benefit in support of those coveted accomplishments in just a few minutes a day.

The vagus nerve is 80% sensory, and supplies information to the brain as to the status of the organs and intestines. It is a motor nerve for the pharynx, soft palate, and larynx, and provides subcortical control for the trachea, bronchioles, esophagus, gall bladder, pancreas, small intestine peristalsis and heartbeat. It helps these systems return to balance if over-stimulated in times of hyper-arousal (fight/flight/freeze in a stress response), and is being considered as a treatment for anxiety, depression, PTSD, and some psychiatric disorders. (Sigrid Breit, et al., March 2018)[48]

Some helpful "remedies" for vagus nerve imbalance besides manual therapy include the aforementioned yoga, meditation, music, tai chi, Hanna Somatics, singing, and chi kung. There has been so much anxiety in recent years that many articles, webinars, and videos have surfaced recommending ways to reduce anxiety by stimulating the parasympathetic response (rest and digest) in the nervous system via the vagus nerve. Due to its many locations and connections, you can understand why the breath, singing, and exercises that focus on the center of gravity, and anything that settles the heart can also help relax the entire system using this key (wandering) cranial nerve.

Whereas parasympathetic—'rest and digest'—innervation arises largely from the sacrum and brain stem (via cranial nerves), sympathetic innervation stems from the thoracic and lumbar regions of the spine.

Visceral/somatic interactions can often create irritation in an organ or gland when the corresponding spinal segment is compressed or imbalanced, and vice versa, which is why we focused on posture earlier. These nerve pathways are also activated by the stress response, which is why the things that help settle the mind and body are beneficial for many systems.

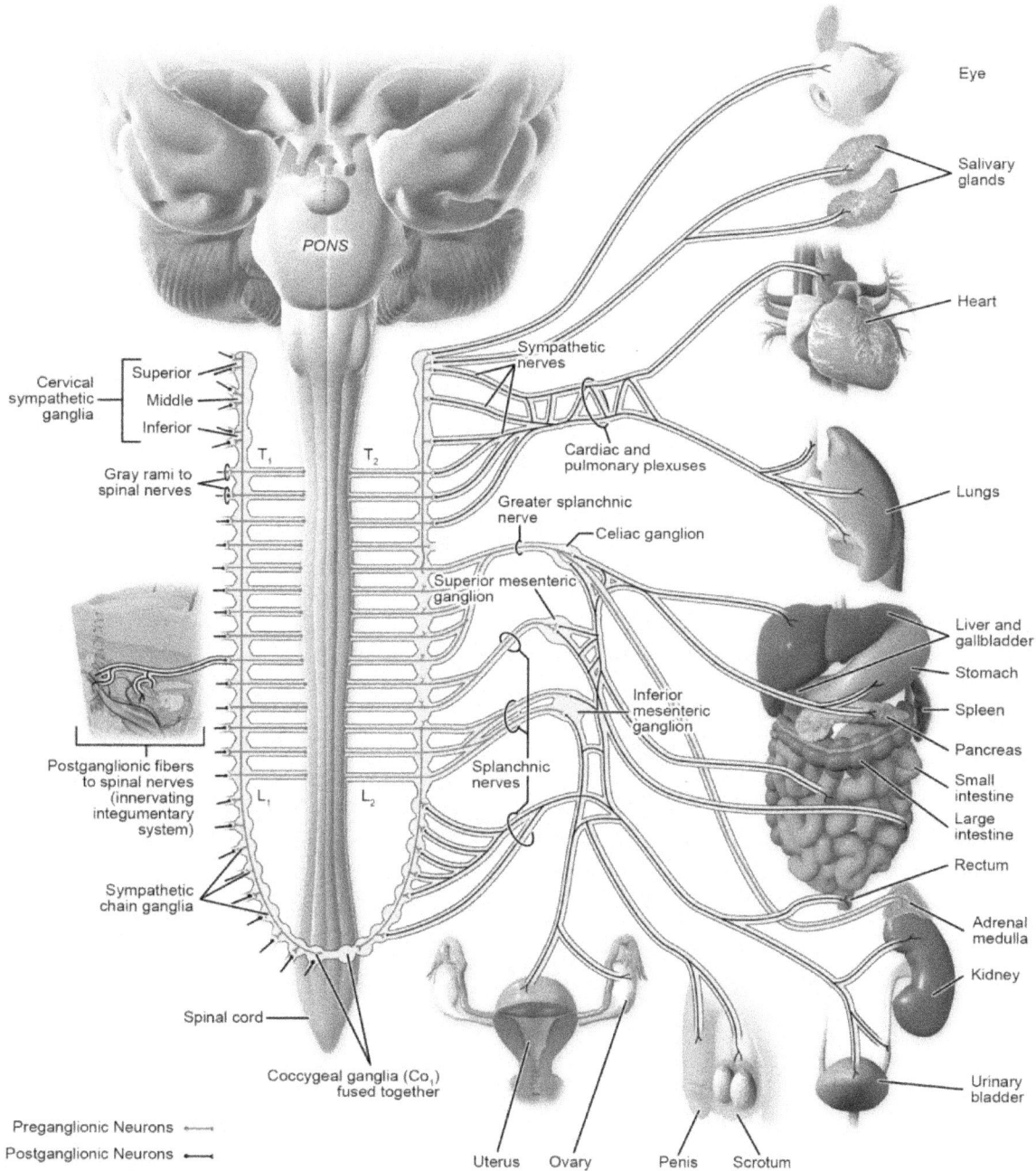

Fig. 3.13 - Sympathetic innervation of the internal organs and glands
Courtesy of Creative Commons Attribution 3.0 Unported

ONE SKY

The brain in the heart

Recent studies show that the heart has its own memory. This fact came to light after inadvertently finding heart donor recipients displaying new preferences and impressions from their donors. It is now believed that some of these memories are stored in the "intra-cardiac nervous system." (Hashim, Albayanti, and Nazal, *Heart Memory and Feelings*," Heart Transplantation, 12 January 2023)[49] These authors believe that neurotransmitters are the medium of transfer of information between neurons, and that there are multiple forms of cellular memory.

There hasn't been a new estimation of the numbers of nerve cells in the heart since 1991 when Dr. Andrew Armour, MD, PhD, declared that there were at least 40,000 "neurites." At that time Dr. Armour stated that the heart deserves to be labeled a "brain in its own right." Not only do these sensory neurites sense heart rate and pressure, but hormonal and chemical information are "*translated into neurological impulses by the heart's nervous system and sent from the heart to the brain through several afferent pathways. These pathways enter the medulla in the brain stem.*

> "*These signals have a regulatory role over many of the autonomic nervous system signals that flow out of the brain to the heart, blood vessels, and other glands and organs, but also cascade up into higher centers of the brain where they influence perception, cognition, and decision making.*" (Madure," *Neurocardiology: The Brain in the Heart*," June 15, 2008){50} Researcher Ali Alshami believes that the numerous interconnections of the brain and the heart—neurological, biochemical, biophysical, and energetic—and the fact that the brain regions that modulate pain are involved, suggest that the heart is also a modulator of cognitive and emotional pain. (Alshami, "*Pain: Is It All in the Brain or the Heart?*," Current Pain Headache Report, 2019 November 14; 23(12):88){51}

Anil Rajvanshi reports that emotions actually control the pace of contractions within the heartbeat. He states that the electrical output from the vagus nerve inputs into the AV and SA nodes of the heart and are reflected in the ECG patterns. It has also been revealed that the heart's magnetic energy field is about 500 times stronger than the brain's (Salem, 2007)[52}, and that it can function as a 'carrier wave' of information that can enact coherence for the entire body. (McCraty, Bradley, & Tomasino, 2004) This coherence has been found to enhance mental clarity, creativity, and positive feeling states. Professor Omar Salem states that, "*The heart is now seen as a highly complex, self-organizing information processing center with its own functional brain that communicates with and influences the cranial brain via the nervous system, hormonal system, and other pathways.*"

Improving disc and associated vertebral segment motion

There are endless benefits to aligning, awakening, and integrating these key structures of the midline. There are also several ways to approach these structures and improve their function. It always helps to remember that you're contacting several tissues, nerves, vessels, bones, and efficient little cells that are listening to your contact and creating the best change they can at the time. They can be more specific when you are being more specific. An atmosphere of ease is also helpful, as it sets the stage for more intricate modifications at some point if needed when there is less "noise" in the system.

Review the layers of intercostal muscles in Figure 1.11 and all the various directions in which they are offering support. Notice the largely vertical, but at times diagonal muscles of the back of many sizes and shapes that will also play a role in the changes that happen. Within those structures is a fascial matrix that is so malleable that it will change from moment to moment depending upon the movement being introduced. For these reasons, when approaching the ribs we will incorporate a few different trajectories so we can test which angle will afford the greatest reset.

Since our somatic pioneers have thoroughly researched the topic, as described in Volume 8, it is clear that there is a direct relationship between the spinal nerve roots that pass by the rib cage attachments and the internal organs (Figs. 3.9 and 3.13). Stubborn places in the intrinsic layers of the paraspinals will often release with gentle reorganization of the ribs, which are easily compressed by all the lifting and carrying we often do. It can be helpful to open the spine more first by doing a few arches and curls, cat/cow, child's pose, downward dog, and the like. If by chance you have a recently damaged disc (Fig. 3.14), perhaps forego this movement.

A recent disc injury will often shift the pelvis off to the opposite side of the extrusion to avoid downloading your weight onto it. Don't try to correct this type of compensatory pattern. Stick with lengthening stretches and decompressing movements for a few weeks.

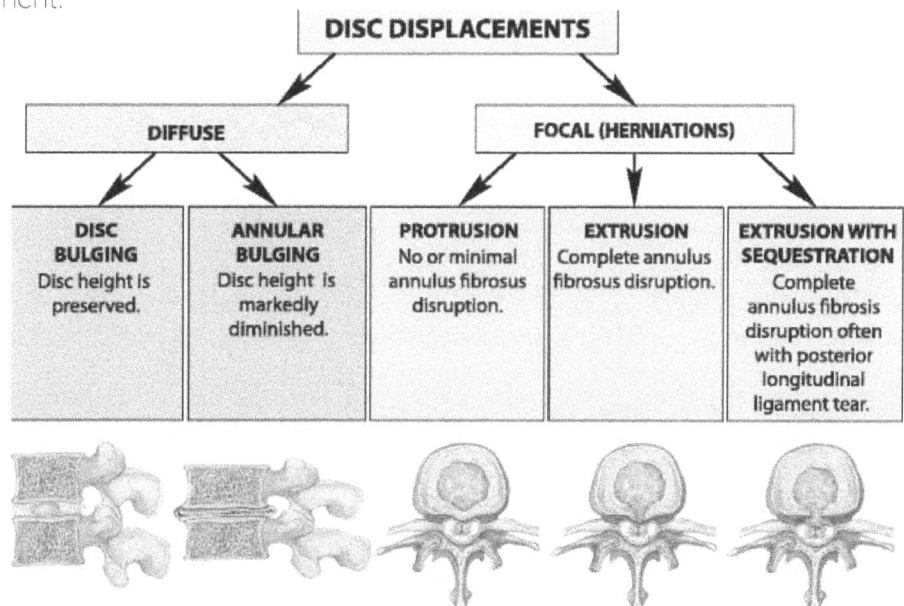

Fig. 3.14 – Classification of disc displacements/injury
Image courtesy of Irina Nefedova, CC BY SA 4.0, via Wikimedia Commons

Rib sequence to improve spinal motion

Rib Release

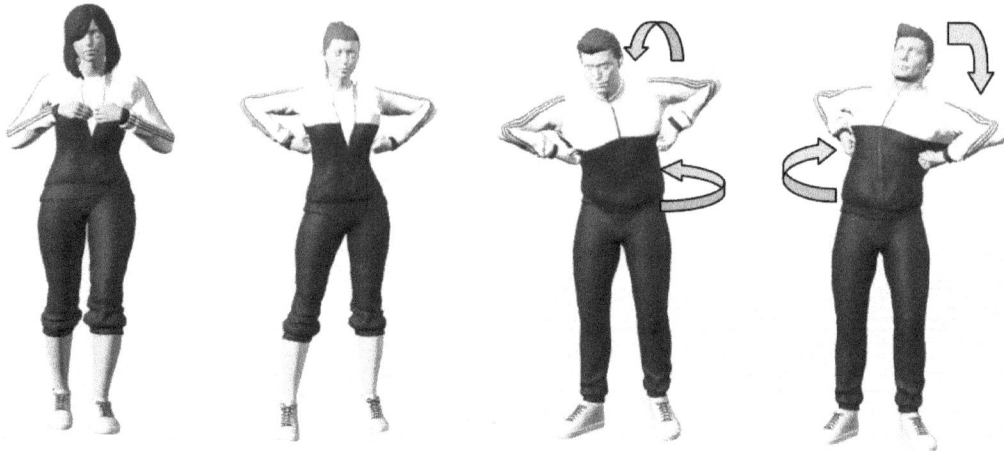

Group 1: Compress, lift, tilt, arch, and curl

With soft fists, place your hands near the bottom of the rib cage. Press in slightly until you feel a tiny motion of yielding in the ribs you're on top of. Very gently lift the skin with your soft (no tension) fists as you slowly arch, then curl your lower back and sacrum.

Move your fists up one rib and repeat until you've gone as high as you can, which is, optimally, to your armpits. Return to the lowest rib (R11, not 12 —the floating rib) and begin again, this time gently side-bending to the right as you ever-so-slightly **lean back** and rotate right as you lift the skin and press in just a tiny bit. Repeat this sequence while bending and rotating to the left.

Next, repeat the above—fists gently lifting the skin as you side-bend and rotate to the right, ever-so-slightly **lean forward** before you being arching and curling as slowly as you can. Move up one rib until you reach the arm pits, then begin again at the bottom as you do this sequence again while side-bending and rotating to the left.

Come back to neutral balanced posture and relax there for a few seconds.

Group 2: Breathe, move, sense, and modify

Place soft fists on the lower ribs and gently press inward slightly. Notice if any section of the ribs feels a little more rigid than another; if it's more resistant to compression. Take a deep belly breath, stretch the skin upward, and notice if one area of the skin is more taut than another.

Arch and curl your low back and sacrum gradually from this hand position, and track the changes in your chest and abdomen, skin and ribs as you do. Exhale and notice the difference in sensations in your body with the out breath. Walk up with your fists to the next rib and repeat.

Inhale and side bend into the tighter side, and rotate very slightly to the right and **elevate** (lift toward the ceiling) your head, neck, and spine as you gently, barely, **lean back** before you arch and curl again. Be aware of any changes that happen in the new position, then exhale and wait a few seconds before changing position again. Move to the next rib and repeat on the left side.

Repeat the sequence, making note of any changes in sensation with each new position and action of arching and curling, but this time **lean forward** after you side bend and rotate.

Group 3: Breathe, sense, listen, and modify

Place your soft fists on your lower ribs and compress them very gently just a tiny bit, being aware of the parietal peritoneum and the tissue fields just on the surface of and just inside the ribs. Pause a few seconds as those fields adjust themselves to the pressure. Inhale, notice the further adjustments as you lift your spine and head toward the ceiling and slowly arch and curl. Then exhale, side bend, and rotate slightly to the right before **leaning back** an inch or two. Notice how your system responds to each new position, and wait for it to adjust, take up the slack, and resettle in a new space. Walk up the thorax rib by rib until you reach the armpit. Repeat this sequence on the left side of your body.

Come back to center in a neutral baseline posture and feel the status of your body after those movements. Compare the felt sense of the right side to what you notice on the left. Once again, be aware of the elasticity of the ribs on the left as you side bend to the left, and notice the changes in the ribs and soft tissue around them when you inhale, rotate slightly, arch and curl gradually, and **lean** just a tiny bit **forward** into flexion. Adjust any place that feels uncomfortable until it feels comfortable based on the feedback from your body.

Come back to center and press your soft fists gently up the ribs to see what feels different to you in their elasticity, and in the sensations or mobility of your spine. Recall which areas of your spine and ribs were calling for modification, and which positions were the most helpful to make those modifications. Notice whether your posture is easier to maintain in a balanced way. If something feels heavier or less supportive of an easeful, neutral stance, make a mental note of where it is and continue to monitor it during the next exercises.

Exploring parasympathetic connections with the brain and thymus

Aspects of the forebrain, midbrain, and hindbrain were developing at the same time as the foregut (mouth, larynx, and esophagus), midgut (stomach, liver, duodenum, and hindgut (excretory system) were developing. Each and all are vulnerable to dysregulation and dysfunctions as a side-effect of chronic stress, illness, injury trauma, or over-exertion without self-care. Scientists used to think that the thymus, which has a great deal of influence in training T-cells for the immune system, atrophies after adolescence and turns to fat (Fig.3.15). They now know that it remains active throughout life, and that people who have it removed are much more vulnerable to diseases and death within 5 years. (Shmerling, Harvard Health Publ, 2023)

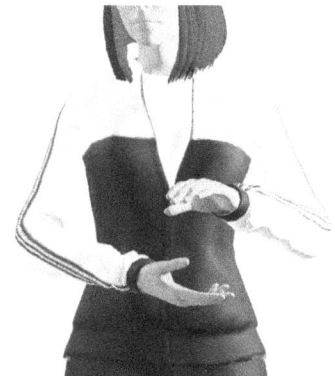

ONE SKY

It takes a few minutes to bring a calming reset into these systems that are intimately connected to the nervous system. You can do this with your own hands. Start by rubbing your hands together a few times to get them warmed and "charged" up, then form a small ball between your empty hands, feeling the energy pulse and tingle between your hands. Try this with these parasympathetic sequences.

What you'll be holding and why it's important for your body

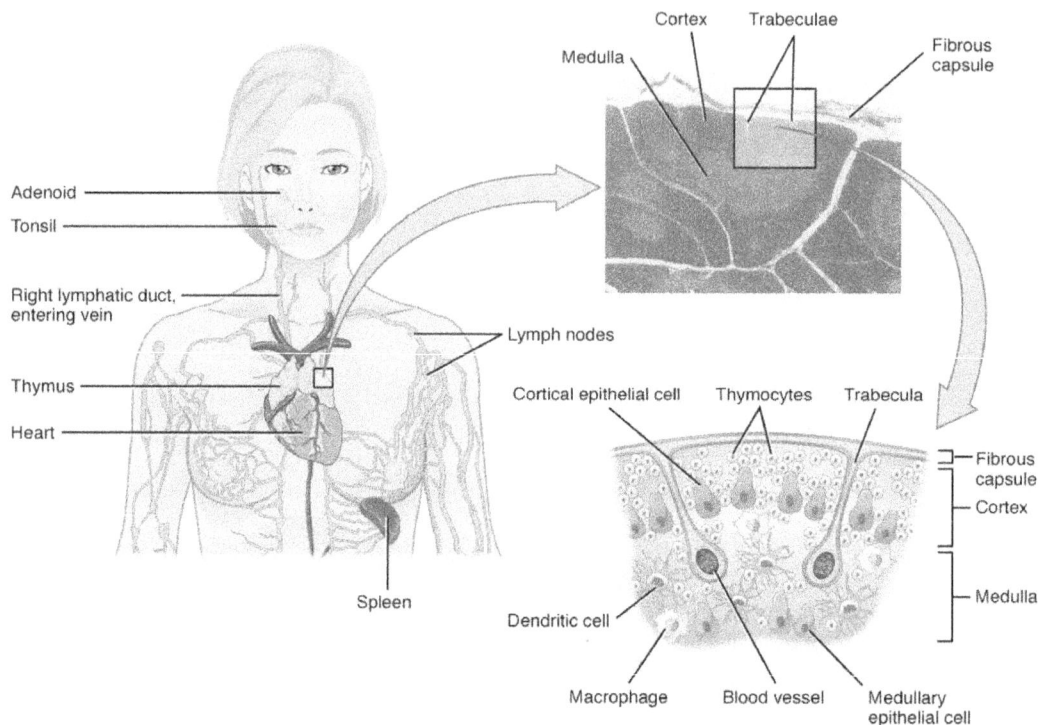

Fig. 3.15 - *Anatomy of the Thymus Gland, aka the 'High Heart'*
Courtesy of OpenStax College CC BY 3.0, via Wikimedia Commons

The thymus gland is significant in many ways. Like the appendix and tonsils, it was thought to be expendable until it was removed in certain autoimmune disorders like myasthenia gravis. Studies have subsequently shown that in fact autoimmune diseases can increase with a thymectomy. Some researchers have found it to remain active even after 100 years of age. (Kameron A. Kooshesh, et al., 2018) Apparently, surgeons will sometimes remove it to gain easier access to the heart, since its proximity can in some people be in front of the heart. It's considered to be part of the immune system, although it's also a gland that produces hormones like thymopoietin, thymulin, thymosin, thymic humoral factor, and small amounts of melatonin and insulin. (Lynne Eldrige, MD, July 11, 2023)[53].

It helps the body identify and fight off foreign invaders, but it can also attack the body if it becomes dysfunctional. Both T-cells and B-cells help fight pathogens and play a role in adaptive immunity, but just the T-cells are trained and released by the thymus. Stress, emotional distress, viral, bacterial, or fungal infections and cancer drugs can all put a strain on the thymus and trigger atrophy. In children, it can at times regenerate itself, but after a certain age the damage or shrinkage remains. Dr. Eldrige reports that malnutrition, starvation, alcoholism, and constant physical strain can also be factors that shrink this gland and weaken immunity.

On the other hand, things that enhance thymus function include carotene, zinc, vitamins A, E, C, B6, and selenium (Murray and Nowicki, 2020). It has also been suggested that the herb thyme supports the thymus, and it is no wonder since thyme has many benefits for immune function. There is also evidence to support the fact that regular exercise benefits T-cell function and adaptive immunity. Some say that there is an additional chakra or energy center there and that it is a source of higher, more divine love; hence the term, "higher heart." In each and every case, it's helpful to know what's underneath your hands when you make contact with your body. It's important to realize that you are having an impact on these systems and upon your well-being.

What's behind your hand at the base of the cranium?

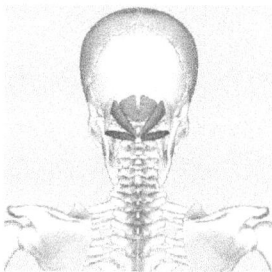

Fig. 3.16 – *Muscles that attach at the occiput Courtesy of CC Attribution BY-Share Alike -2.1 JP*

The occiput is a major intersection for blood flow to and from the brain, for cerebral spinal fluid flow, sensory and motor nerve impulses to and from the brain, along with the origin and insertion of several muscles (Fig. 3.16) and ligaments. Deeper inside the skull is home to the cerebellum, a key organizer of movement and the occipital lobe, which can set off the sub-occipital muscles if working at a computer too long. The visual cortex helps organize spatial relationships, visual memories, depth perception, object or face recognition, and color. The cerebellum also influences balance and coordination, but has connections to emotional parts of the brain as well (Fig.3.19). Recent studies have the cerebellum involved in the perception, recognition, forwarding, and learning of emotional information. (Camilla Ciapponi, et al, 2023)[54]

Ciapponi finds that in recent decades studies are reporting that the role of the cerebellum has expanded to include higher order functioning like emotional and cognitive processes that "substantially contribute to the generation of experiences and the control of emotional states," similar to the way in which it compares intention with execution for motor behavior. The cerebellum also plays a significant role in visual acuity and efficient eye movements. (Beh et al., 2017)

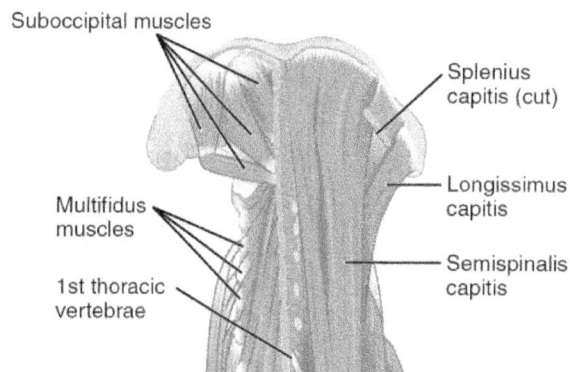

3.17 - *Sub-occipital and neck muscles that are influenced by contact at the occiput OpenStax, CC BY 4.0 via Wikimedia Commons*

One Sky

What's behind your hand at the forehead?

The prefrontal cortex and the front of the brain have executive functions that other areas of the brain listen to for instructions and corrective feedback. A stressful childhood or a bump on the head here can create poor emotional or impulse control, a lack of consideration for the consequences of one's actions, attention deficit disorder, and other cognitive issues. It can also shape personality, decision-making, mood, and motivation. Apparently, some brain scans have shown very little prefrontal activity in the brains of murderers. There is a lot of interaction between the frontal lobes and many other areas of the brain, the heart, and belly brain, so when you place your hand there, you're also contacting and influencing other areas.

There are a few dense layers that can produce a response to touch even before you reach the actual brain, which is quite soft. On the surface or outer layers, you may notice a release in soft tissue of the scalp, the periosteum or dura (Fig. 3.18). Even the cranium (skull) itself can release intraosseous (within the bone) compression and begin to open, soften, widen, and change shape. What you may notice is a change in behavior, in balance and coordination, flexibility, dexterity, posture, temperament, clarity of vision, or attentiveness and focus. Reduced tension and a sense of pervasive calm may act as feedback that you have affected the brain itself.

Keep in mind while making this and every contact with your body, that it is an alive, sensitive and responsive, intelligent organism that is open and curious about whatever you are doing. It is generally compliant if not happy to make whatever adjustments it has at its disposal to make itself and you more comfortable.

If you allow your hands to be soft and relaxed when you touch, more can be sensed. Your hand is just as much of a receiver and transmitter as any other part of your body if not more, as a great deal of sensory and motor space in the brain is dedicated to the hands. Approaching the following explorations from this perspective will enhance, inform, and deepen your experience.

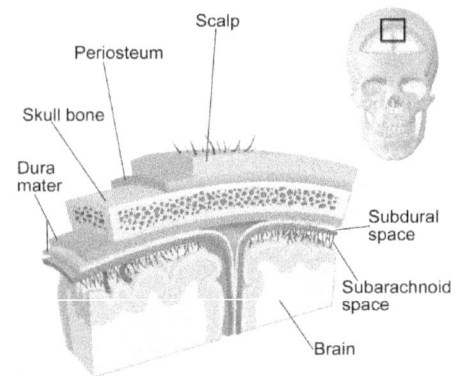

Layers covering the Brain

Fig. 3.18 – Initial layers you'll make contact with when touching your forehead
Courtesy of Creative Commons Attribution 3.0 Unported

Parasympathetic Manual Therapy Sequence 2

Group 1: Make conscious contact

While standing in your best neutral baseline posture, find the most comfortable position for your hand that will be on your sacrum. Close your eyes before placing the other hand at the back of your head, just above your neck for 10 breaths.

Then move that hand to your forehead just on or above your eyebrows for 10 breaths. Next, place the moving hand just above your heart and below the collar bones, which will be directly over the thymus for 10 breaths. Then shift to a gentle placement on your heart for 5 breaths.

Although simple, these hand placements are very potent because they awaken and connect key systems in your system, potentially initiating rebalancing in many systems that are on circulatory, neural, endocrine, organ and musculo-skeletal levels.

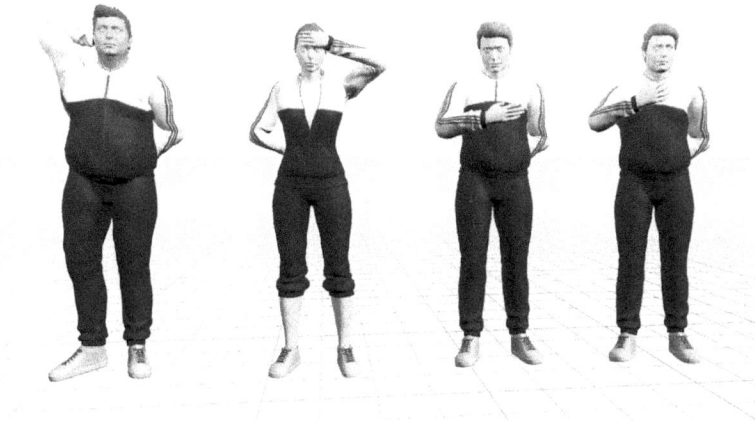

Group 2: Connect, breathe, and sense

Find the most ease in your stance while placing the hand on your sacrum that fits most comfortably there. Cup the other hand at the back of your head just above the neck, and notice the shape of your skull. Does one side feel a little different than the other in shape, position, density, or size?

Take a deep breath, hold it for a few seconds, and notice what changes in between your hands. Exhale, hold the exhale and wait a few seconds again. Did anything change in your skull or sub-occipital muscles? Do you feel any blood vessels (heartbeat)? Breathe normally for a few seconds and reset your hand on the thymus.

Notice the sensations and intrinsic movements that may arise on the anterior and posterior of your system, as well as deeper within. Breathe normally and be aware of which changes occur throughout your system with this hand placement. After your system settles, move your hand down to your heart and monitor the responses from your body.

Group 3: Sense, pause, breathe, follow

Replicate the instructions for Group 2 with the following modifications: When you sense the body adjusting according to the contact with your hands, and with the addition of a sustained inhale or exhale, pause and wait for the body to complete its reorganization before your next breath, or your next hand position.

Notice the local responses right where your hands are, the activation that happens between your hands that can create shifts in muscle tension, mood, energy levels, or global organization. You may even sense changes in the skin, membranes, or fascial layers.

Wherever they occur, follow the motion that your body produces with these shifts with your attention and your hands.

What you'll potentially be contacting beneath the skull

Due to the interrelated functions among the structures you'll be contacting, there will be ways in which you'll access multiple areas of your cranium and brain regardless of where your hands are placed. Both frontal and cranial base regions are connected to limbic (emotional) and reward (dopaminergic) systems, autonomic functions, as well as sensory and motor feedback loops.

The frontal lobe (Fig.3.19) is much more involved in decision-making, memory, language, personality development and expression, voluntary movements, overall cognition, and executive "control" over behavior and social interactions. Both are key areas to make contact with in order to help integrate changes or to help settle the system. A useful exploration to apply, which may come naturally to cranial therapists, would be to feel into the third ventricle, or into the seat of the hypothalamus.

There is a different type of reset that can happen by contacting an area that may be considered to be a more metaphysical realm of influence. Although it has often been considered to be the Ajna chakra that sits near the center of the brain relative to the pituitary and pineal glands, the description of its location is more closely related to the anterior (and posterior?) commissure. The posterior commissure sits just in front of the pineal gland. This area functions as a nerve plexus that is exactly where the right and left nerve fibers cross, where one side shares input from the other side of the brain hemisphere and body, and it does the same throughout the length of the spinal cord while resting at the top of it.

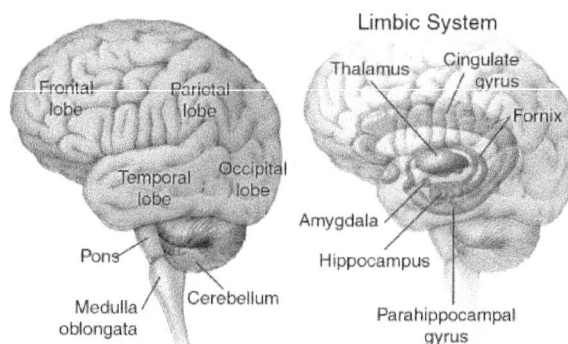

Influenced by hand placement (not shown – pituitary, pineal glands near the front and back of the thalamus respectively)

Could the Ida and Pingala channels-the two nadis of Kundalini yoga that flank the Sushumna or central channel-be the carriers of the 'neurotrophic factor' that the somatic pioneers spoke of, allegedly delivered by the nervous system? Are they part of the Primo Vascular System that nourishes the entire body—only recently discovered to have an observable form? The anterior and posterior commissures also work with memory and emotion, both of which can be stored within nerve cells. All of these possibilities are worth exploration into how they relate to overall well-being in ways we're still beginning to understand. Whatever the overlap may be between energetic and anatomical structures, just know that the center of the deeper brain region can bring great ease and peace.

Chapter 4
Explorations that Connect the Three Brains

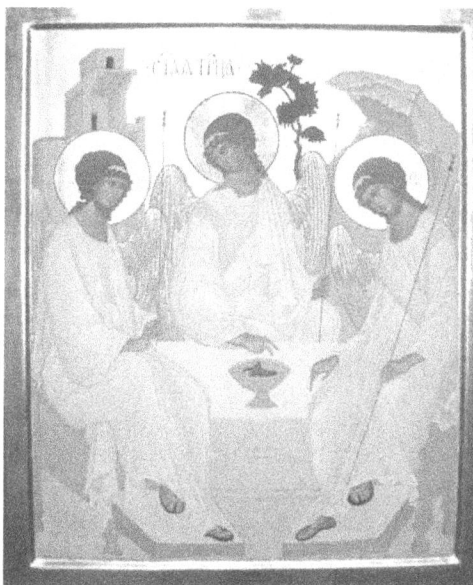

Courtesy of a group of people, CC0 via Wikimedia Commons

We are once again going to address the major forms of communication within the body because of where they're located, and how they were derived embryologically. These three systems—the cranial brain, the heart brain, and the belly brain—are given brain status due to the numbers of nerve cells and neurotransmitters they contain, and the fact that they receive and transmit signals using the central nervous system. They are in constant contact with one another and are easily influenced by one another in directions that can either increase or decrease balance on many levels. Therefore, anything we can do to ease a source of agitation or tension in any of these systems and enhance their unimpeded flow of coherent information will be beneficial in many ways.

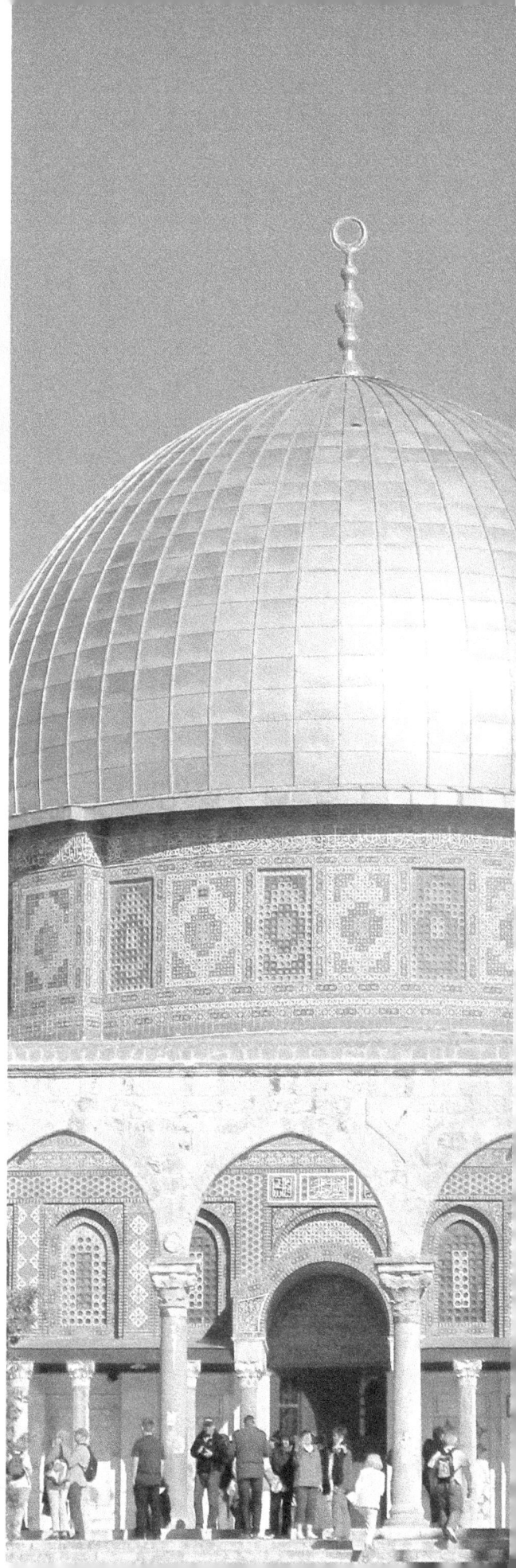

We discussed the cranial brain in detail in Volume 8, and we covered several aspects of the heart brain already in this text. The enteric nervous system in the gut deserves a little more attention before we proceed into the explorations that connect them. The Cleveland Clinic states that, *The gut-brain connection is complex and bidirectional. Signals pass both ways between your digestive system and central nervous system, and health or disease in one can affect the other. Key players in this connection include your enteric nervous system, your vagus nerve, and your gut microbiome.*

A long list of common ailments springing out of this connection's cross-talk when stress dominates the interaction includes various

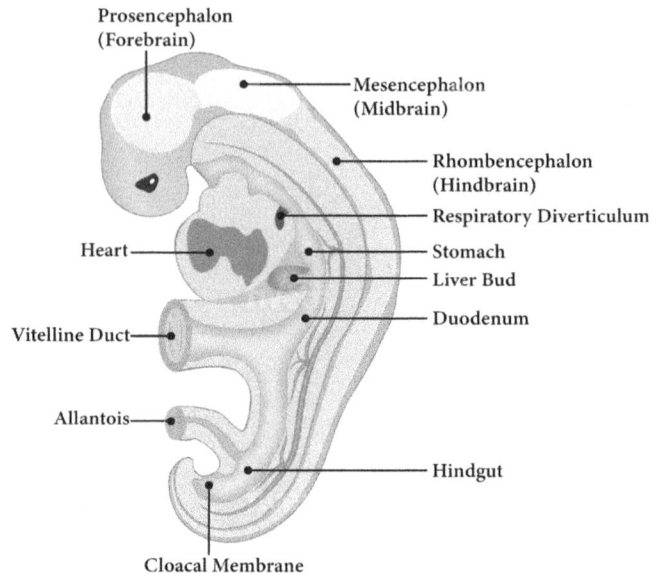

Fig, 4.1 – *Formation of the gut tube in the 28-day embryo*

gastric disorders, anxiety, mood disorders, chest pain, chronic fatigue, and obesity. (Cleveland Clinic, "The Gut-Brain Connection," 2023)[55] A great deal of the enteric nervous system is in the lining of the gut tube, where approximately 168 million nerve cells reside.

The gut tube and enteric nervous system

The gut tube is one of the first structures to be derived from the endoderm in the embryo's first month of life. Among other things, the cloaca—or primitive anus—is in front of the area you'll make contact with at the sacrum, making it even more influential as a primary messaging structure for the entire body. Marilla Carabotti, et al. reports that, *"The gut-brain axis (GBA) consists of bidirectional communication between the central and the enteric nervous system,* **linking emotional and cognitive centers of the brain with peripheral intestinal functions."**

She goes on to say that these connections include neural, endocrine, immune, and humoral (body fluids) links. (Carabotti, et al, 2015).[56] There is a growing body of research happening in the ability of diet and/or specific probiotics that improve the functionality of the microbiome to assist in balancing mood disorders, and even autism. (Ribeiro, et al., 2022) The lungs, also derived from the endoderm, began as a small bud alongside the gut tube so it also has a direct line of communication with it via the immune system. Perhaps that's where the phrase, "inner skin, outer skin" comes from in Chinese medicine. Due to the microbiome they share, the nasal tube, gut tube, lungs, and skin are all connected and reflect imbalances in one another.

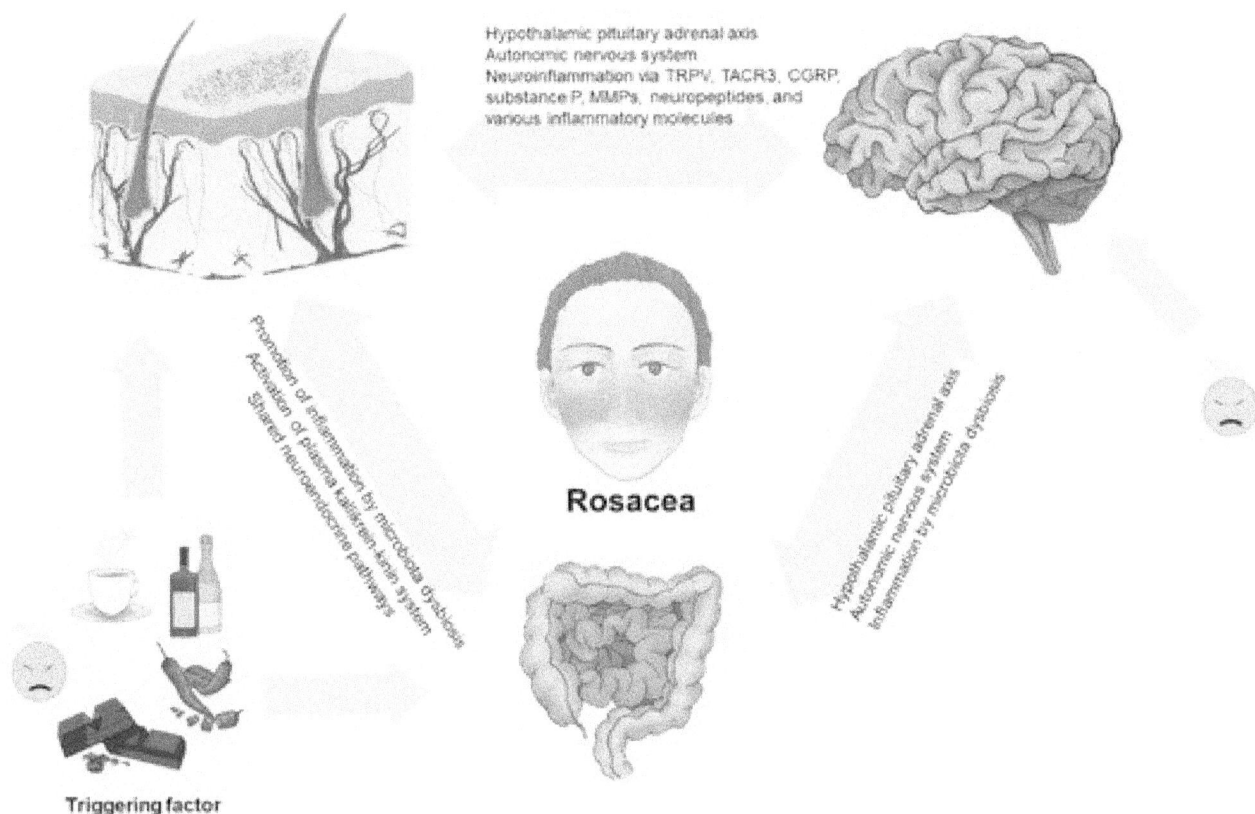

Hypothalamic pituitary adrenal axis
Autonomic nervous system
Neuroinflammation via TRPV, TACR3, CGRP,
substance P, MMPs, neuropeptides, and
various inflammatory molecules

Rosacea

Triggering factor

Fig. 4.2 – *Gut/Brain/Skin Axis*
Courtesy of Creative Commons Attribution 2.0 Generic

The skin in particular can manifest symptoms of dysfunction or distress in any of the other related systems (Fig. 4.2). Considering outbreaks in the skin from this point of view is an important shift in perspective. These relationships are bio-chemical, and therefore potentially corrective at the source. It's possible that myofascial techniques are effective because they make use of the skin as a significant transmitter of information throughout the system. Remember that in the embryo-where the body begins forming itself-the mouth, esophagus, trachea (foregut), lungs, stomach, liver, pancreas, gall bladder (midgut), intestines, and anus (hindgut) are one long inseparable tube. This is most likely why people vomit or experience bouts of diarrhea during periods of overwhelm or intense stress.

They remain deeply interconnected in structure, function, signaling pathways, and processes. Touch, which is how we will be signaling these structures, immediately interacts with receptors that transmit information to and through the peripheral and central nervous systems including the brain. As discussed in depth in Volume 8, the skin is a powerful mediator of information for the entire system and can be a reflection of issues in the intestines (Fig.4.2). The skin also transduces biomechanical input through movement, which can benefit every system.

ONE SKY

Touch is a requirement for well-being

One aspect of touch that hasn't been focused on but is gaining momentum is the requirement of touch for mammals, including humans, to develop cognitively and socially. It is currently a topic of research regarding neurodegenerative disorders as well as autism. (Jenkins and Lumpkin, 2017)[57] These and other researchers concur that input from the several types of touch receptors in both superficial and deeper layers of the skin are transduced into electrochemical forms of information that can influence any system in the body including the organs and viscera, which have millions of receptors in its skin/epithelium (Fig. 4.3) and numerous hormones, peptides, and neurotransmitters that communicate with the brain. There is a growing body of evidence that **healthy brain function is directly related not only to touch on the skin, but to microbial balance in the gut.** (Chen, 2021)

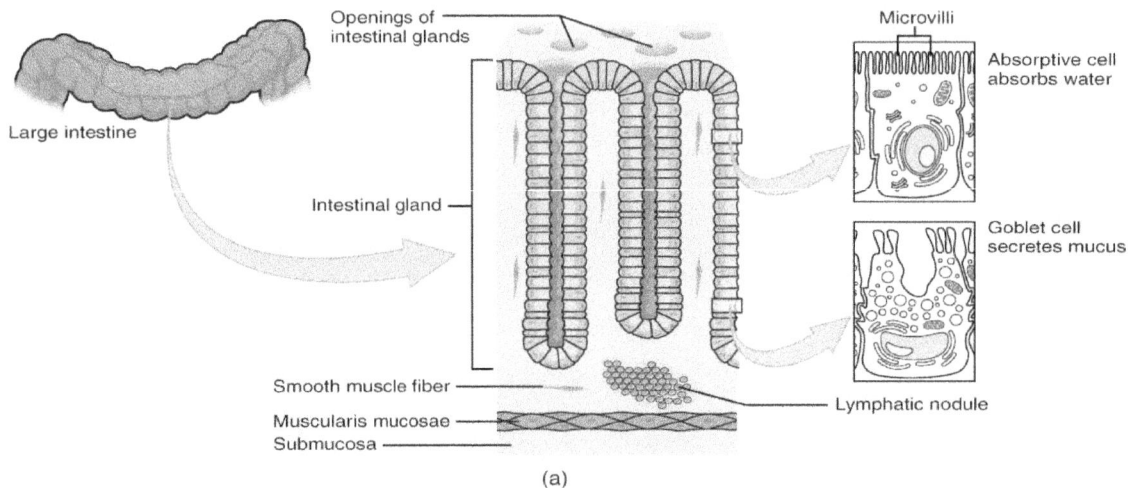

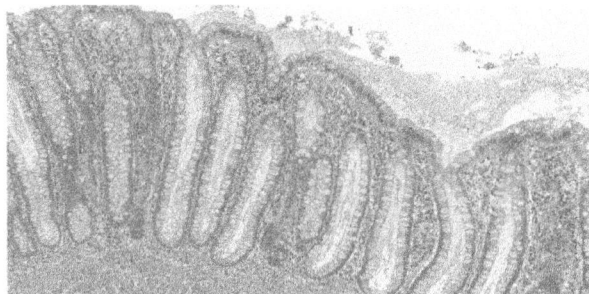

Fig. 4.3 – *Histology of the Colon Courtesy of OpenStax College, CC BY SA 3.0 via Wikimedia Commons*

Casey Henley asserts that there are receptive fields for each of the receptors in the skin, and when they are activated, these fields become awakened and sensitized. When more than one area is contacted, then **the entire field between these points becomes activated** and awake. This is why making contact by pairing areas that are already inherently connected by the germ layer they are derived from becomes even more potent in their ability to create an acknowledging reset. Stretching the skin enhances the potential for self-correcting even more. (Casey Henley, Foundations of Neuroscience, 2023)[58]

Group 1: Linking the Wires

Rest one hand on your belly while the other hand remains comfortably on your celiac plexus/solar plexus. Remain in this position for 10 breaths.

Leave the hand on your belly and move the other hand up to your heart and pause there for 10 breaths. Repeat after placing the moving hand on your forehead.

Group 2: Track sensations as you breathe

Rest one hand on your belly brain while the other hand rests on your celiac plexus. Notice any changes in the abdominal cavity or lower back in the tissue fields, fluids, joints, or energy flow. Breathe into your belly with even inhales and exhales. Notice if you feel a sense of connection between your hands.

Settling the Brains

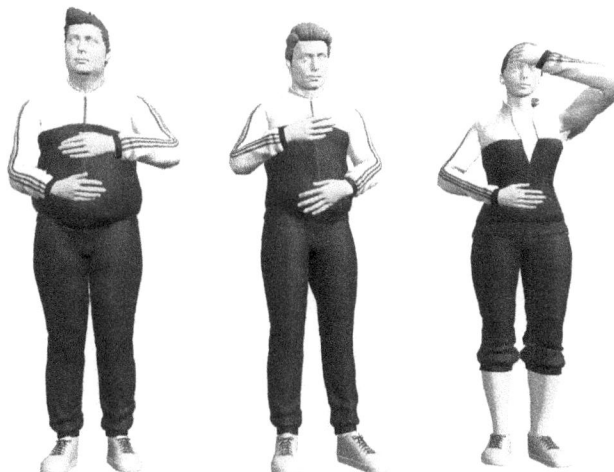

Move the hand on your belly slightly to see if there are different responses that happen when your hand is on the transverse colon versus the ascending and descending colons or the small intestine.(Fig.4.3). Do the viscera move when your hands move?

Come up to the heart area with that hand on the solar plexus, and have the sense that your anterior hand is feeling those structures that are a few inches deep, in front of the spine. Adjust your hand placement slightly and notice what changes in your body's response. Repeat with that hand over your forehead.

Group 3: Sense, monitor, pause for response, and follow

Replicate the sequence that's described for Group 2, with the difference being that as you sense how the body responds to each hand position, wait for the response to complete its adjustments before moving to another hand placement.

At times, as the tissue and fluid fields are changing under and between your hands, the body will glide them into a slightly different position as if to point out the next place that could use some reorganizing. Some places move more slowly than others or take a bit longer to recognize where your hands are, so wait a few seconds until it completes its response.

Groups 2 and 3 Integration:

Take some breaths, holding the inhale and exhale a few seconds with hands by your sides. Notice if your energy and posture are more effortless, how your weight feels on your feet, and up through the skeleton.

There are similarities between the inner skin (intestines) and the outer skin, even in their structure and function. Each has a layer that protects, and a layer that metabolizes, transduces, and transmits information. There's also a layer that has immune function (Fig. 4.3) along with an inherent connection to the nervous system. Each has a microbiome that is a significant regulator of the health of the inner and outer skin, both of whom have a bidirectional relationship with the nervous and endocrine systems, which is why transdermal patches work. They also can reflect imbalances or agitation therein.

The celiac plexus is also a significant nerve center that lies deep in the upper abdomen and has self-regulating qualities prompting some to call it a little brain in its own right. It innervates the lower esophageal sphincter, the stomach, spleen, kidneys, upper small intestine, liver, gall bladder, and pancreas. (Candal, Reddy, and Samra, 2023; Jan Vascović, MD, 2023) It has parasympathetic (Vagus nerve), sympathetic (greater and lesser splanchnic nerves), as well as nociceptive fibers.

This plexus, or group of nerve ganglion, sends messages to the brain from the foregut and midgut that either promote or inhibit digestion, depending on whether the sympathetic or parasympathetic fibers are being activated. It transmits sensory input from these areas as it descends from the T12/L1 area of the spine while wrapped around the aorta from the associated celiac, superior mesenteric, aortico-renal, inferior mesenteric, and superior hypogastric ganglion (Fig.3.13). Meditators and yoga enthusiasts will already be aware that the main nerve plexuses in the body correspond to a few main chakras or energy centers. This could be why there's evidence of physiological benefits from both of these practices.

Exploring connections between the extremities and the core

These last sets of practices exploring connections with the parasympathetic plexus using the sacrum and other significant nerve and/or communication centers are supremely calming and balancing for the system. It's a great way to begin or end the day as well as to start a movement or exercise sequence from a calm, neutral place in your body. The next sets of movements will explore releasing the influence of the extremities upon the core, or on the midline.

It's important to remember that whatever we do with our arms and legs, hands and feet, is being supported and stabilized by the core, the thorax, and the center of gravity. For this reason, many types of cumulative tension become paired with distal (farther away) areas of the body. Sensing into those relationships by pairing them and feeling the pull between them will serve their release and reorganization; their mutual reset. There are other movement possibilities that are more complex interweavings, which we'll also explore.

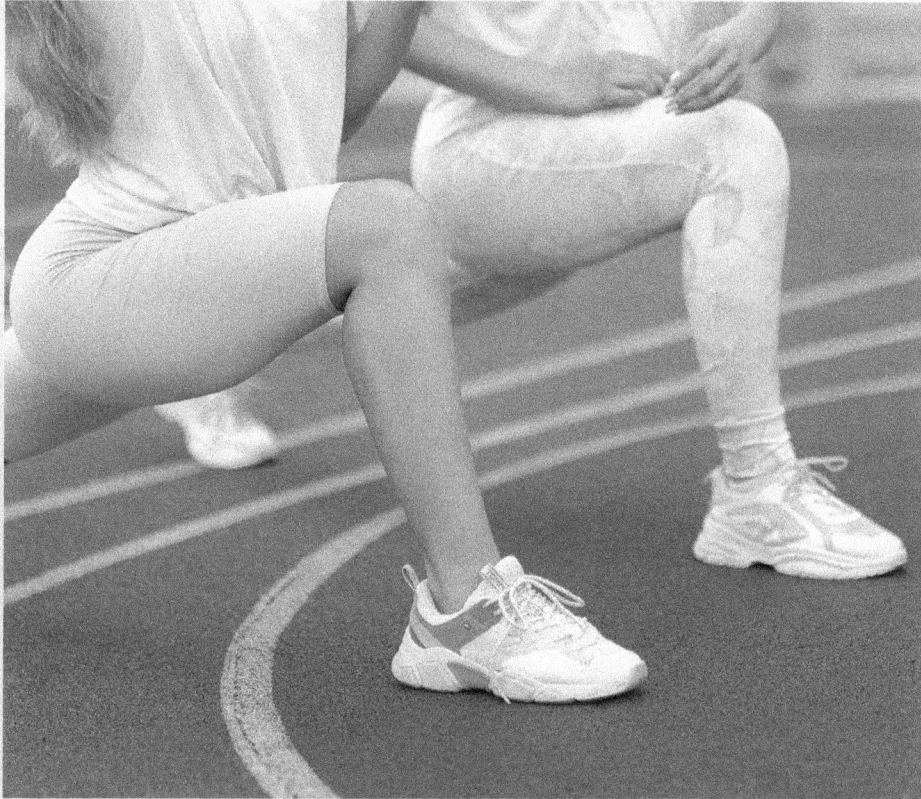

Section 3

Movement and Manual Therapy to
Release the Midline Brains

> Sutherland hypothesized that within a nerve trunk the highest known
> element is formed. Like the information is formed within the potential
> of a coaxial cable, Information can be carried in this space.
>
> *Dr. R. Paul Lee*

Let's begin with a movement you're already familiar with and add somatic principles to it.

Modified Lunge 1

Group 1 is welcome at any time to experiment with the recommendations included for the other groups. In particular, the breathing aspects may prove useful for the increased openings and relaxation in your body.

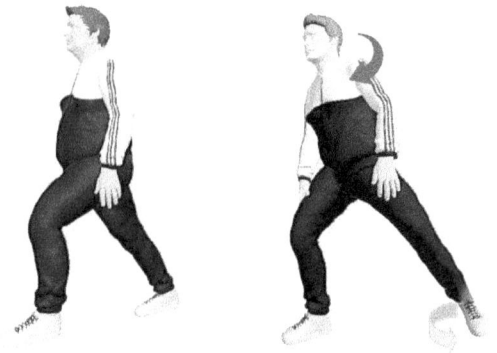

Group 1: Lunge with variations

Place one leg forward and bend that knee while extending the other leg behind you in a moderate lunge position. Don't let the knee in front go beyond your toes. Only lean forward and extend as far back as feels comfortable for your feet, ankles, knees, and hips.

Keeping your back straight initially, lean forward a bit more as you extend the back leg a bit farther behind you in small increments. Place the other leg in front and repeat the gentle movement.

Take a deeper stance if your body accepts it easily, and lean away from the extended leg. While in that position, slowly rotate the hip and foot of the extended (back) leg in the opposite direction that your upper body is leaning. Change legs and repeat.

Group 2: Sense, breathe, and adjust

Lean into a gentle lunge position and feel where the most tension is as you lean forward and extend the back leg. Notice any catch points in and around the pelvis and groin areas. Breathe in and lift your chest as you lower the heel on the back leg if possible. Exhale and rotate your hips slightly in the direction of ease, or of less resistance.

Inhale and slowly pivot the back foot so the toes are more outward and the hip and leg also rotate externally. Exhale along the length of that leg. Switch legs and repeat.

Inhale and rotate your torso in the opposite direction of the back leg very slowly as you notice which areas of the leg have the most influence on the ability of the pelvis to feel freer. Exhale as you lean and rotate forward and back a fraction of an inch in order to open the tissue fields in the abdominal area.

Group 3: Sense, listen, pause, and adjust

Follow the instructions for Group 2, but pause a few beats in each position in order to allow time for the system to make its own modifications in the area.

There may be more than one area that responds to the new position, so wait until the entire body has had a chance to review and adapt to the changes. Breathe into your belly while you wait. Take up the slack produced by your body's response by opening or deepening the stance.

During the slight rotations of the torso and back leg, locate and return to the position that produced the most tension, then soften the stance slightly, breathe, and extend again with the leg. Lift the chest and rotate more to see if your body was able to open more to accommodate the stance. Switch legs and repeat.

Modified Lunge 2

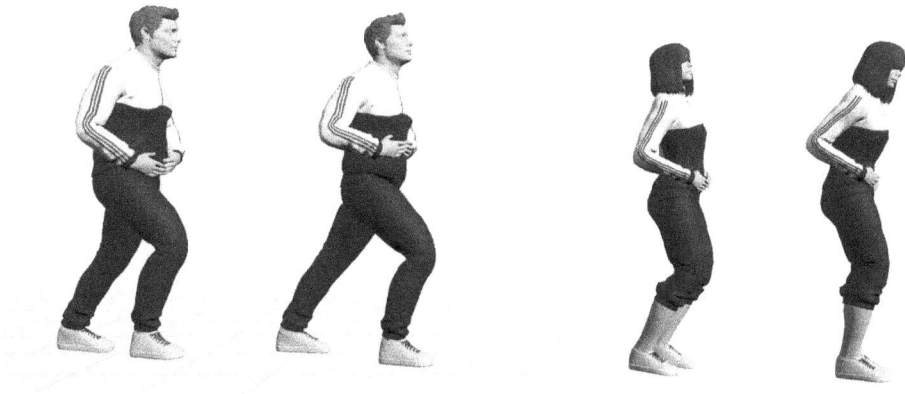

Releasing the visceral brain from the surrounding tissue fields

Group1: Posture, hold, stretch up

Assume your best balanced posture while in the lunge position and place your hands gently just inside the pelvic bones (Fig.3.13).

Gently press in and up, cupping your lower abdomen in your hands as you extend your back leg slowly away from your hands that are above the groin area; just above the inguinal ligament. You may be able to contact the iliopsoas muscle in this area. Repeat this action when the other leg is extended behind you.

Raise your hands a bit higher, placing them just below your rib cage, and gently press in and up again. Simultaneously, lift your chest and lean back slightly while extending your back leg. Switch legs and repeat.

Return to a neutral stance and cup your lower abdomen again, this time doing a slow, gentle arch and curl with your lower back a few times.

Group 2: Move, sense, breathe

Follow the instructions for Group 1 for a basic sequence. Notice where the lines of tension are under your hands and gently modify the angle of your leg that's placed behind you to optimize the release of the widest area of sticky tissue.

Move the legs forward and back, knees bent a little or not at all; in closer to the center or farther out to the side, toes point in or turned out more as you inhale. Hold for 3 seconds, then exhale at each position. Switch legs and repeat.

ONE SKY

During the arches and curls, leave your legs the width of your ribs, and move as slowly as you can through the range of each vertebrae, breathing more deeply when you sense a stiff section. Hold the inhale as you arch, curl, do tiny rotations each direction, and exhale. Feel each motion all through the spine if you can.

Group 3: Move, sense, listen, wait

Follow the instructions for Groups 1 and 2 with these additions: The tissue under your hands will begin to shift as soon as you press in and lift, and again as you extend the leg back. Wait for these changes to complete as you breathe into your hands.

Take up the slack provided by the tissue as it opens and allows your hands in deeper, and allows for your leg to extend farther back with ease.

Feel the difference along the entire side when you switch legs, and allow your body to make changes as it notices your hands. Compares the sides before you begin. Adjust your torso until you feel the connection under your hands with the back leg.

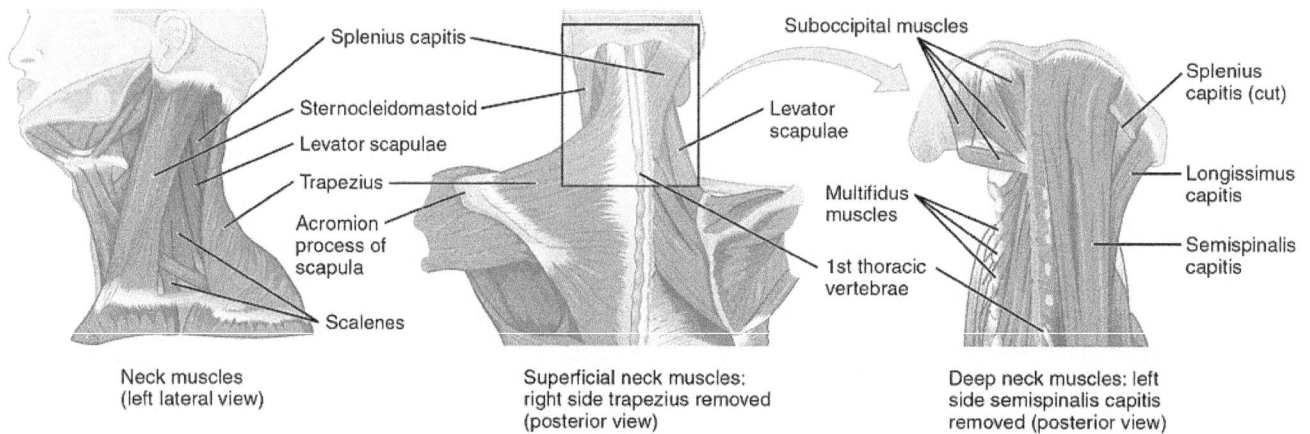

Fig. 4.4 – Illustration of muscles that are greatly influenced by the use of the arms and hands and often pull on the spine
Courtesy of OpenStax, CC BY 4.0, via Wikimedia Commons

Peripheral muscle groups that influence the heart brain

You will find that the center of gravity is working to hold the foundation steady as you use your arms and hands throughout the day. They wind up becoming, just like the lower body, wired into many of the membranes, muscles, and fascia around the heart, lungs, and organs under the diaphragm. Very often, to achieve a full release of tension in the upper back, neck, spine, shoulders, and abdomen, the arms will need to open to allow an exchange of information up through the neck and thorax/torso. Being very powerful flexor muscles, along with the fact that we're in flexion for most of the day, the pectoralis and biceps will need to be addressed due to being intertwined with the use of the hands.

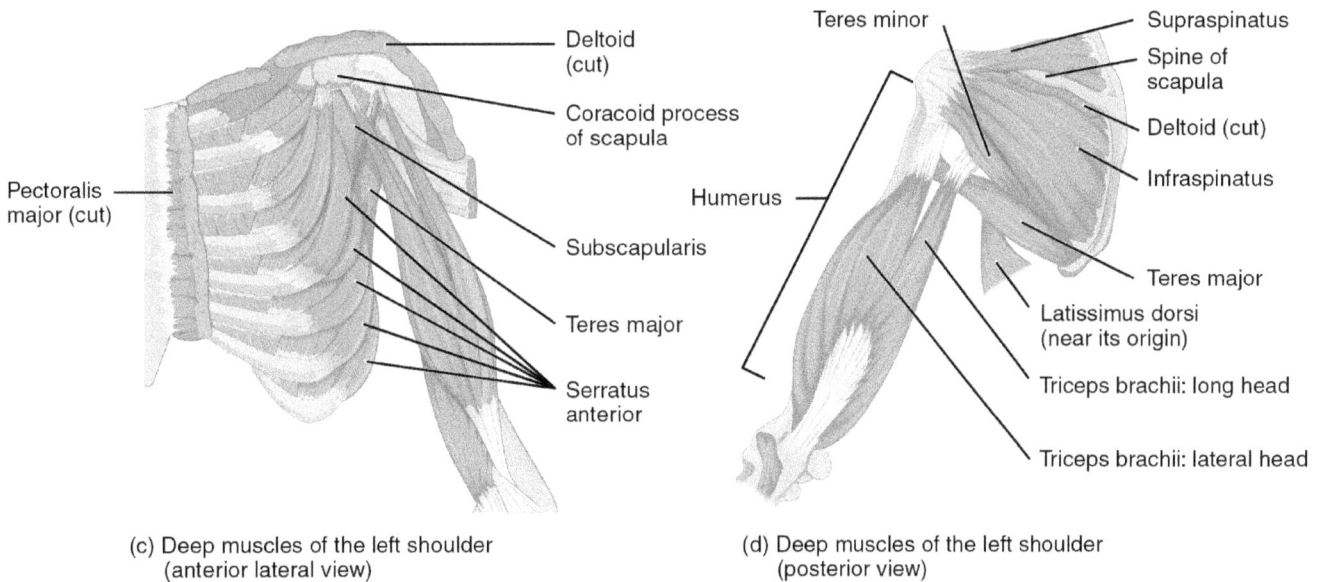

Deltoid (cut)

Coracoid process of scapula

Pectoralis major (cut)

Subscapularis

Teres major

Serratus anterior

Teres minor

Humerus

Supraspinatus

Spine of scapula

Deltoid (cut)

Infraspinatus

Teres major

Latissimus dorsi (near its origin)

Triceps brachii: long head

Triceps brachii: lateral head

(c) Deep muscles of the left shoulder (anterior lateral view)

(d) Deep muscles of the left shoulder (posterior view)

Fig. 4.5 – Illustration of muscles that pull on the cervical spine with the use of the hands
Courtesy of OpenStax, CC BY 3.0, via Wikimedia Commons

As you can see, the numerous muscles in the arms, neck, and shoulders are angled in multiple directions to facilitate a wide range of motion in each of the joints, but particularly the neck, shoulders, and wrists. This means that the tensions accumulating in these areas will have formed themselves along numerous angles, perhaps further compounded by connective tissue matrices. Therefore, let's begin by releasing some of the sticky or stiff areas in the retinaculum - or membranes that secure the tendons and vessels coming down the arm as they enter the hand (Fig.4.7). There are also several small carpal bones that tend to become compressed with work involving repetitive motion (Fig.4.6).

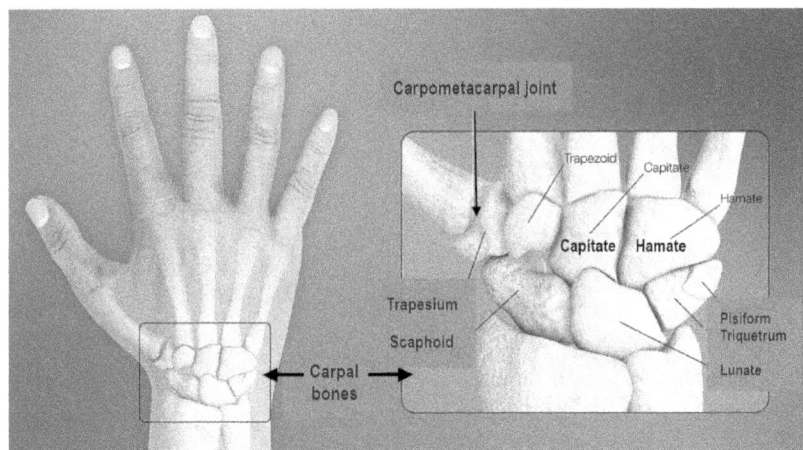

Carpometacarpal joint

Trapezoid

Capitate

Hamate

Capitate

Hamate

Trapesium

Scaphoid

Pisiform

Triquetrum

Lunate

Carpal bones

Fig. 4.6 – Carpal bones of the wrist
Courtesy of scientificanimations.com, CC BY-SA 4.0 via
Wikimedia commons

ONE SKY

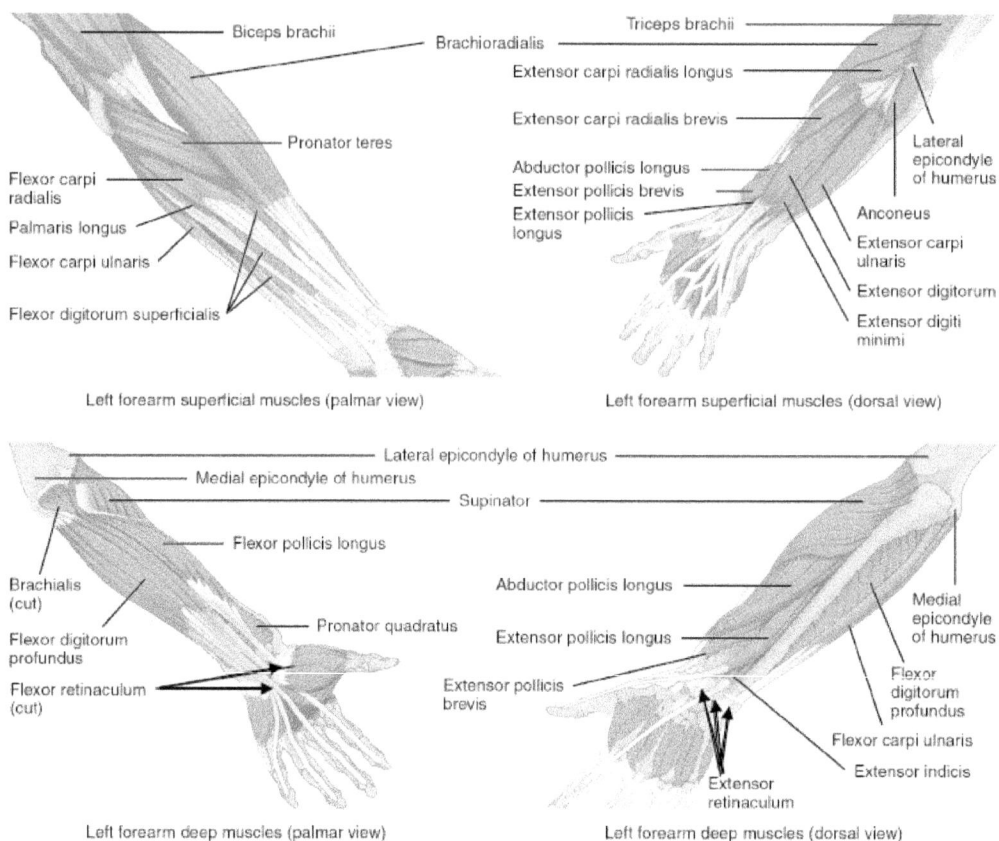

Fig. 4.7 – Illustration of muscles of the forearm that influence the shoulders and neck along with blue arrows pointing to where the (horizontal) retinaculum sits on the wrist
Courtesy of OpenStax, CC BY 4.0 via Wikimedia Commons

Releasing the forces from the upper extremities on the heart brain

This simple motion will help release any stickiness above or below the retinaculum and possibly between the ligaments and tendons in the area so you can more easily free up the muscles in the arm. With a firm yet gentle grasp, roll your hand around the wrist in both directions, taking notice of the direction that feels easier, and monitoring the tighter side as it begins to let go. Move up the hand a bit farther, then a bit lower onto the wrist and continue to observe how your hand, wrist, and arm respond. Next, find a wall that is clear from top to bottom, and raise your arm to shoulder height if you can do so comfortably. Extend your hand so that it's at a 90° angle to your forearm and place the palm of that hand flat against the wall, or as flat as you can. Varying the angles of your arm and hand position will access the many different muscles in the forearm that aren't vertical (Fig. 4.7). This way of unraveling the forces up through the arm upon the midline improves posture and opens the flow through the meridians in the arm that affect the heart, lungs, and intestines.

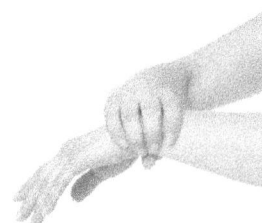

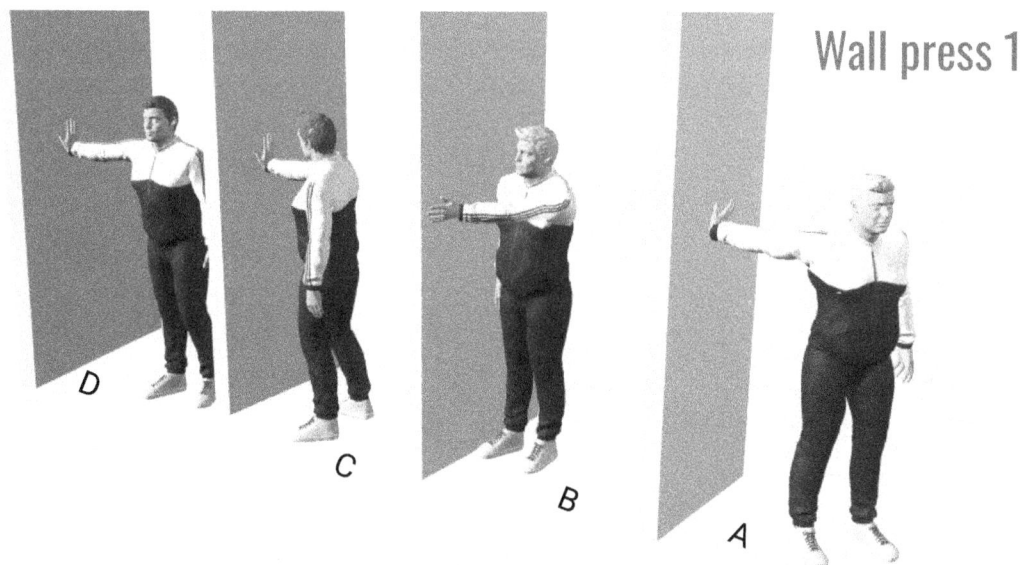

Wall press 1

Group 1: Rotate hand and body positions

While your palm is on the wall with fingers pointing toward the ceiling (D), slowly rotate your body toward your arm, and then away from your arm. Gently, gradually spread your fingers then bring them back together 3 times in each hand position. Repeat with your fingers facing forward (B), then backward (A), going only as far as you can without pain or strain.

Group 2: Move, breathe, and sense

Follow instructions for Group 1, adding a deep belly breath at the outset of each position and hold for 5 counts. During the last spread of your fingers in each position, exhale and hold for 5 counts. Notice what happens all the way up the arm, neck, and shoulder with each arm and hand position, as well as with your breath.

Group 3: Move, listen, breathe, and sense

Follow the instructions for Groups 1 and 2, but wait and let your body finish responding before changing hand positions. Take up the slack when the muscles and connective tissue let go and soften, possibly enabling you to straighten the arm a little more, or to flatten the palm a bit more with less resistance. Be aware of whether your system lets go more with the inbreath or with the out breath. Notice how your posture has changed after completing this sequence.

Releasing forces from the chest and arms on the pericardium

Wall press 2

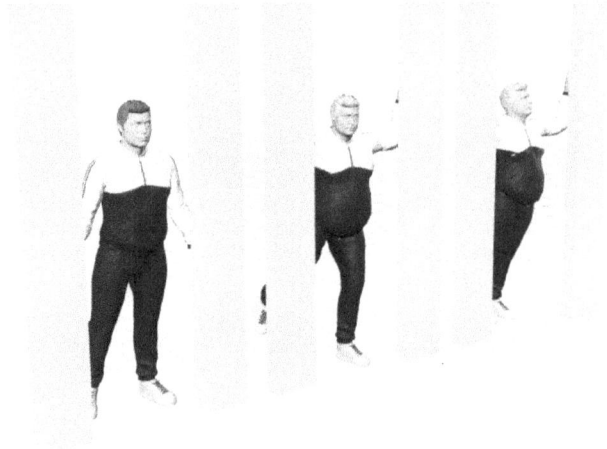

A - Arms low, feet apart   B - Arms high with a lunge   C - Arms high, feet together

Side note:

Now that the most distal (hands and arms) tensions have been more neutralized, we can come in more proximal in search of restrictions in the chest in relation to the shoulders. Find the most comfortable position for your arms to be supported by a door frame. If you have any shoulder issues, you can have your arms lower without the elbow bent (A).

Only lean as far forward as you can easily do without feeling strain in any joint or anywhere in your body. Avoid double-jointed positions by keeping just enough tone to support them not over-extending. Use your whole body for each position, not just your arms and chest. i.e. tighten your back and legs just a tiny bit for support.

Group 1: Move slowly, change gently

With your arms in a position on the door frame that feels comfortable for your shoulders, slowly lean about 3 or 4 inches through the door opening, and hold for 2 breaths.

Then push yourself back to a neutral position and repeat the lean with a slight rotation of the torso to one side to reach some different fibers of the muscles. Push back and rotate slightly to the other side.

When you lower your arms, pay attention to whether the exercise had an effect on your posture. The pectoralis major and minor muscles are used consistently throughout the day and will benefit greatly from this movement.

Group 2: Move, breathe, sense

Take a deep breath, exhale, and gradually lean through the door frame, noticing the affect on your rib cage, the muscles in your upper back, and the lengthening in the abdomen.

Be aware of which areas of your body respond to the breaths that you take, and test it to see if it feels better to move forward into the stretch on the inhale or the exhale.

Push back to your original position and rotate slightly to one side, noticing which fibers are more ready to open up. What happens with your shoulder blades? Push back again, rotate to the other side and repeat. Explore how your body responds to breathing into your chest versus the belly.

Group 3: Move, breathe, sense, pause

Follow the instructions for Group 2, and at the end range of your leaning through the door, exhale and let your body have a moment to adjust and reorganize. What's happening in your diaphragm, pelvis, or spine?

Have you noticed an area of your body that has revealed an obvious connection to whatever is happening in your chest and shoulders, such as your belly or hips?

As you breathe, allow the space for those areas to unravel in relation to one another at end range, and as you make slight adjustments along the way.

Wall press 3

Arms lowered with
neck rotation

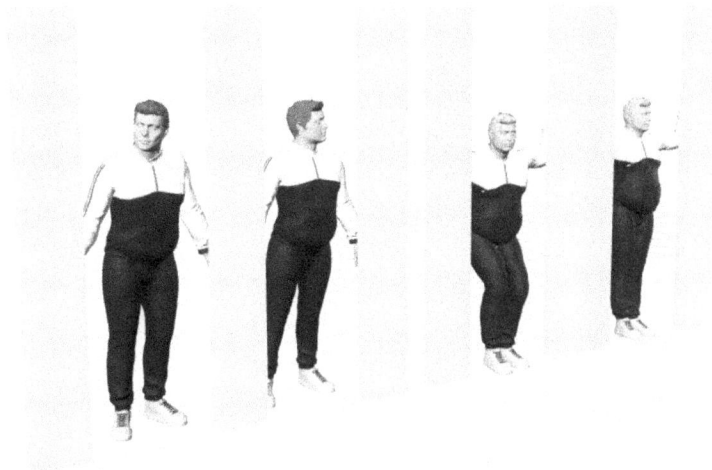

Bend and straighten
your knees

Group 1: Move gently and slowly

This type of movement affects the intended areas—the back, chest, neck, and shoulders—by moving a different area that's connected to them through function and by shared fascia fields.

With arms lowered, mostly straight and palms directly on the door frame, lean forward slightly while gradually turning your head from side-to-side. Does either side pull into the shoulder when you turn? Leave your forearms where they are, gently bend your knees, then gradually drop your body straight down as if you're about to sit. Slowly move up and down three or four times making sure that your shoulder joints are comfortable.

You will be able to contact actions of both the anterior and posterior shoulder girdle muscles during this movement, along with a few rotator cuff muscles. Be sure not to strain. Find a balanced position for the shoulder joint before moving up and down.

Group 2: Add breath and sensory awareness

Follow Group 1s sequences, bring awareness to which arm position in the doorway brings the most neutrality in your chest. Breathe in, notice what the area in between your ribs feels like, and slowly bend your knees. Notice the changes in your entire torso and shoulders with the new position, then inhale, hold for 3 seconds, exhale, and compare the right and left sides.

Which side expressed the most ease with each action? Did both shoulder blades move smoothly? Were there differences in the sensations produced by your forearms, your biceps or deltoids? Stand up again and take note of any differences you feel in the original position before repeating the sequence. When your arms are lowered, does your neck turn more easily in one direction than the other? Does the breath create more ease? Do your collarbones move with your breath?

Group 3: Include listening and waiting

Repeat the instructions for Groups 1 and 2, but after you inhale, wait for the tissue to respond and adjust itself before breathing out. Be aware of the space between your shoulder blades as you breathe, and as you bend your knees. Is there a position for your feet that feels more comfortable for your knees or for your hips? Modify your position for balance and neutral joints as you bend your knees, then breathe in, let the body reorganize, and exhale. Try to identify which areas of your body adjust themselves the most as you hold the inhale and exhale for 3 seconds in each new position. When you lower your arms and rotate the head and neck, try extending and flexing your head just an inch or so to see which position affords the most benefit for them, for your chest, and for your back.

Releasing forces from the posterior torso upon the midline

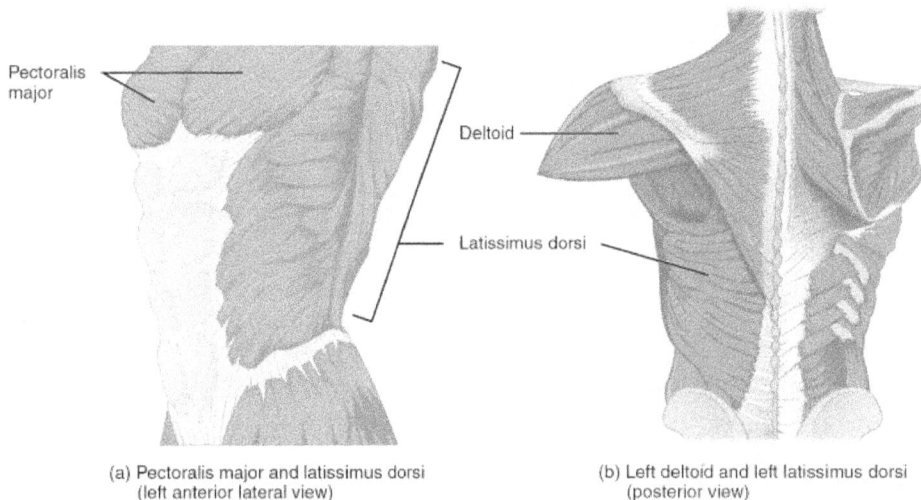

Fig. 4.8 – Muscles that move the upper arm (humerus) *Courtesy of OpenStax CC BY 4.0 via Wikimedia Commons*

(a) Pectoralis major and latissimus dorsi (left anterior lateral view)

(b) Left deltoid and left latissimus dorsi (posterior view)

Wing Work 1

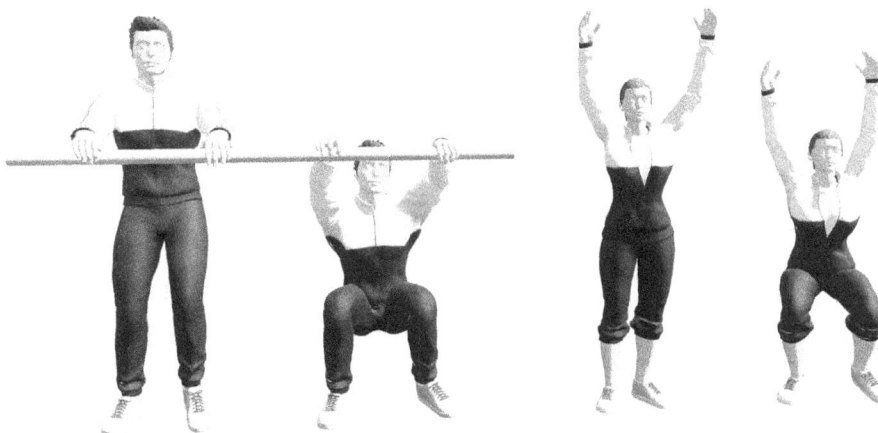

As you grab the bar and bend down, the outer layer of the pectoral muscles as well as the deeper pec minor muscles (Fig. 4.5) will be releasing pressures from the midline in front, which helps the upper back muscles (Fig. 4.4) to also let go.

You can see that the latissimus dorsi runs all the way down to the sacrum, but inserts at the upper inner arm. It also attaches along the spine, as do the lower traps (Fig. 4.8).

They are both very much influenced by the arms and the legs, which is why it's helpful to release them in a movement that includes all of them.

Group 1: Move gently, consciously

While holding onto a sturdy bar in your bathroom or gym, slowly bend your knees as you drop your body down and away from the bar. Stay down for 3 breaths as your lats and lower traps let go.

Pull yourself back up and repeat the movement 3 times, seeing if you can drop down a bit further each time. Then release the bar and raise your arms over your head. Bend your knees again for three breaths and come back up.

Group 2: Add breath, self-sensing

Replicate the sequence for Group 1, with the inclusion of a deep, slow, belly breath as you descend, hold it for 3 seconds as you track the changes in the lats and low traps. Inhale, pull yourself up as you push up with your feet, and repeat.

Stand tall with your arms in a 'Y' position over your head, inhale and slowly bend your knees, monitoring the changes in your sides, lower back, and shoulders as you exhale. Recheck your posture afterwards.

ONE SKY

Group 3: Breathe, sense, and pause

Duplicate the instructions for the other two groups, but after the inhale and change of position, wait for the re-adjustment to complete itself everywhere in your body before you exhale and come up.

You can experiment with rotating your torso slightly with subsequent bends so you catch different fibers of the muscles. Pay attention to whether your back prefers to be slightly arched, flat, or slightly flexed. When your arms are raised, see if turning your feet more inward or outward makes a difference. Check your posture again afterwards.

Releasing forces from the upper and lowers limbs on the midline brains

Wing Work 2

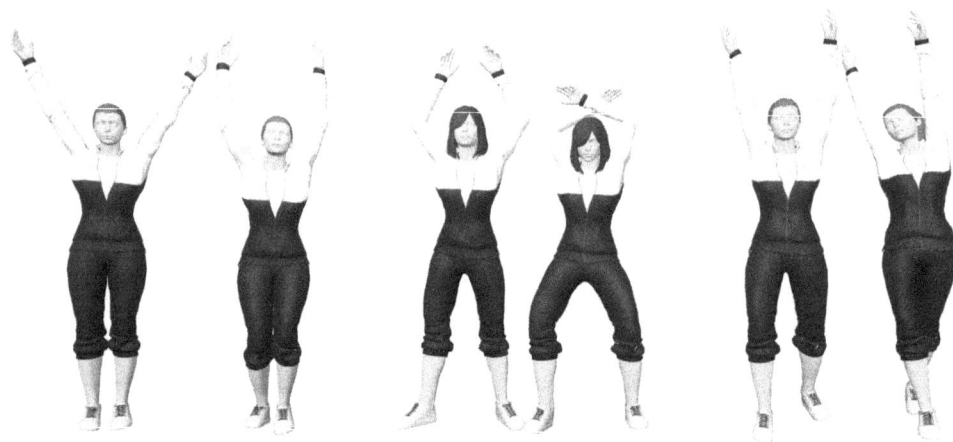

Using variations of the sequences you went through will engage the same muscles in a slightly different way, providing you with helpful information about which combination best suits your body and the release of daily tensions. Activities change, so the movements you'd want to use as a reset will likely also want to change. If you have a torn rotator cuff or frozen shoulder, this series of movements will need to be modified to accommodate what your body feels comfortable with. At no time should you strain or force or override an injury. You can try them with your elbows bent at 90°, 70°, or whatever doesn't create discomfort in the joint.

Group 1: Adjust positions gently

Experiment with a variety of arm positions, hand positions, and stances to optimize the stretch and release you get through your back and shoulders (examples above).

Try a wide stance, a narrow stance, feet straight, feet turned out, knees bent, legs crossed, torso straight, torso rotated, or slight side-bent. Find the best combination of limb placements that gets you the access you need for those hard-to-reach places.

Group 2: Explore, sense, and breathe

Inhale, and slide into each new posture gently with the exhale. Be aware of sensations that feel stiff versus sore versus pinchy or glitchy.

Avoid positions that create the discomfort sensations in the joint by altering the arm or leg forward or back, more inward or wider, or with a different rotation angle until the motion or position feels smooth and easily accepted.

Adjusting a joint/limb position by just half an inch can make a big difference in whether your body feels safe in a new movement.

Group 3: Sense, breathe, listen, pause

Follow the suggestions for Groups 1 and 2, add the aspect of listening to your body's sensations in a way that leads you to make the best adjustments in response. Inhale and listen, move and listen, exhale and listen while following your body's lead and taking up the slack as it releases.

Compare initiating the motion on the inhale versus the exhale, and compare how long to hold each in or out breath to obtain the greatest benefit for your system. Notice when or with which position you can sense the entire lateral line from fingers to feet and rest there a moment or two.

Releasing forces from the hip muscles on the midline and belly brain

We were able to clear some tension from the legs, hamstrings, quads, and psoas during the explorations in the lunge position, hopefully after finding neutral posture. These muscles have a significant influence upon the hips, which are directly connected to the sacrum and midline structures. While standing, it's more challenging to clear tensions in the feet, so we'll address that while supine (lying down facing up). Like everywhere else in the body, the muscles of the hip that move the leg are many and run in several directions. (Fig. 4.10)Therefore, the forces will be transmitted and laid down in multiple angles during our daily activities. These muscles are relatively short, increasingly so as the layers deepen, so they are vulnerable to strain patterns and, as usual, should be approached with care.

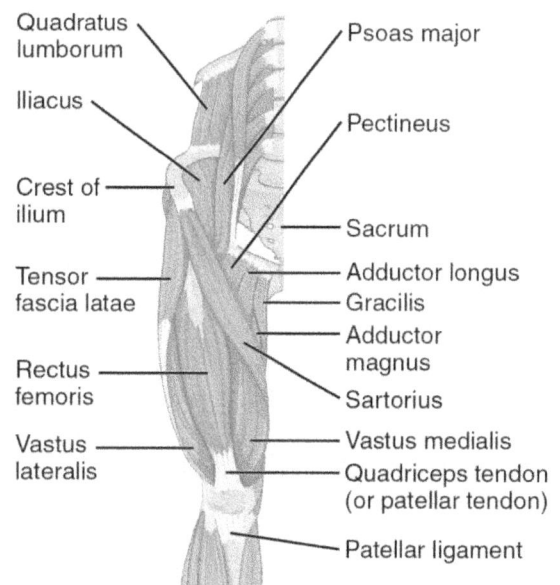

Fig. 4.9 – Anterior muscles that move the hip and leg
Courtesy of OpenStax College, CC BY 3.0 via Wikimedia Commons

Deeper within the hips are many supportive ligaments that surround the joint. (Fig. 4.11) They receive information about joint position, load, speed, and trajectories to transmit to the brain which compares this input with the intention and makes corrections therein. Keeping the joints mobile and free is key to the brain being able to use information effectively to organize muscles and surrounding tissues. When the joints are freer and more balanced, the sensory-motor feedback loops are clearer and more accurate in both directions.

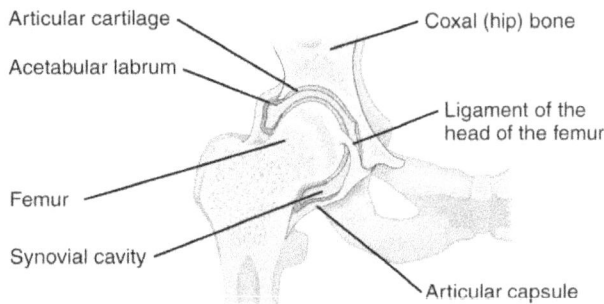

(a) Frontal section through the right hip joint

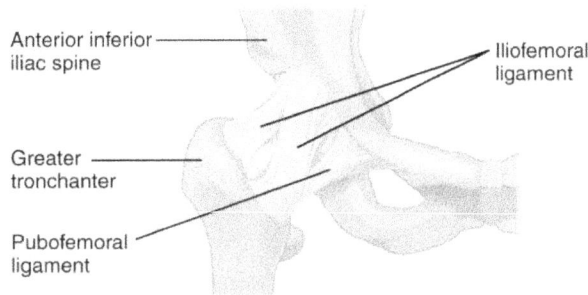

(b) Anterior view of right hip joint, capsule in place

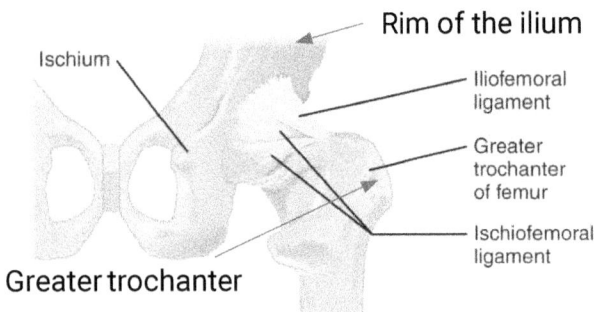

(c) Posterior view of right hip joint, capsule in place

Fig. 4.11 – Cartilage and ligaments of the hip's joint capsule *Courtesy of OpenStax College, CC BY 3.0 via Wikimedia Commons*

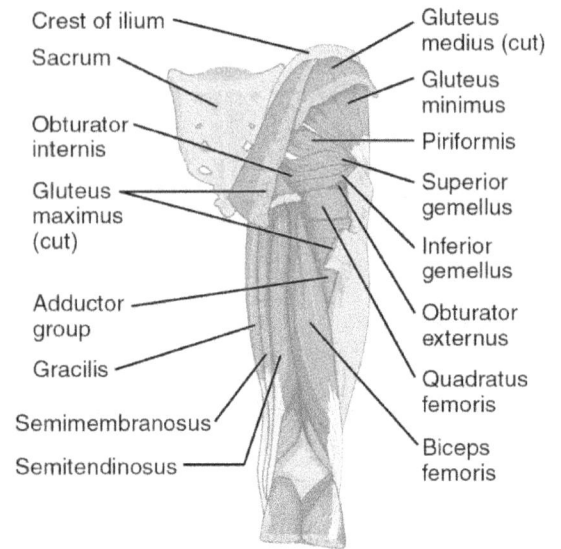

Fig. 4.10 – Posterior muscles that move the hip and leg
Courtesy of OpenStax College, CC BY 3.0 via Wikimedia Commons

Just like any joint, it's important to help them remain open, aligned, and hydrated. Hydration is facilitated as much by the pulsing that happens during movement as by drinking water.

These deeper structures are the ones that will wear down when there are muscular imbalances from use patterns, injuries, from falls, overuse, or adhesions that created uneven patches in the tissue fields.

Lack of information exchange due to stagnation and sedentary lifestyles are just as harmful to these structures as overuse from dance, running, sports, and so on. There are a considerable amount of hip replacements that happen to those who don't exercise or barely work their bodies.

The varied transmissions coming up the chain also leave a myriad of force vectors in the greater trochanter itself. I've found it to be just as helpful to discharge impacts and compression in the bone itself as it is from the joints, muscles, and connective tissue.

Most of us aren't aware of what condition the deeper structures are in, particularly those in and around the joint capsule. Therefore, it's best to have your best elongated posture going before loading the joints with an unfamiliar position or movement.

This next sequence is wonderful for both the hips and for the lower back. It works every time if you position yourself comfortably.

Hula Hips

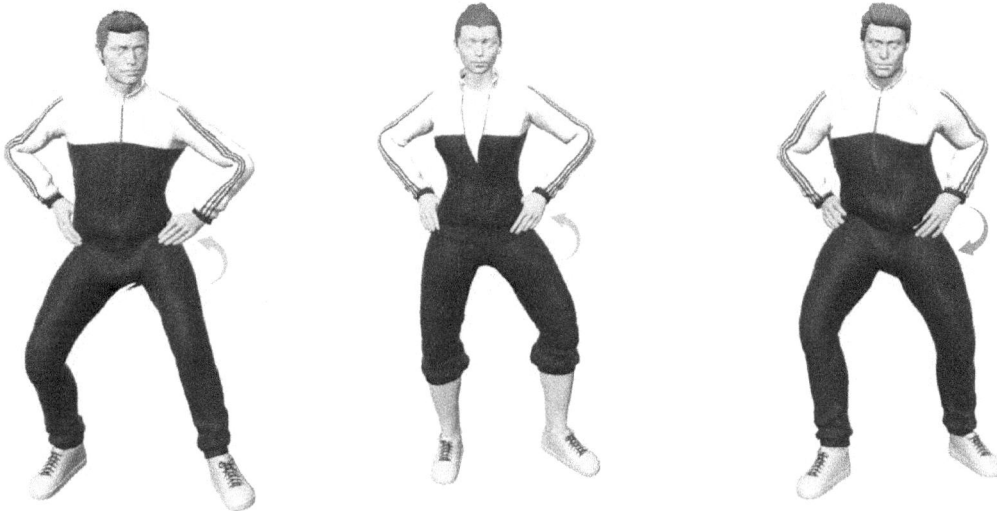

A – The moving leg is forward   B – Both feet are on same plane   C – The moving leg is behind

For this sequence, have your hands on your hips in the space between the rim of the ilium and the greater trochanter (Fig. 4.11); just above the most prominent bone in your upper leg. The leg that will bear the weight, which is the right leg in the provided illustration, is not the side of the hip that will be moving. Take care not to go past your toes with the knee on that side.

Group 1: Move gently and slowly

While leaning back on your right leg, place the left foot a few inches in front of the other one in a wide stance. Rotate the left hip slowly and gently in both directions, then switch legs and repeat.

Bring your feet straight across from one another, keeping your weight on the right leg, and rotate the left hip from front to back in both directions.

Then place your left foot a few inches behind the right and rotate in both directions from front to back (rather than side-to-side.)

Group 2: Sense, place, breathe

Take care in placing your feet so that the right leg feels completely comfortable in supporting the left, and the left leg allows all the joints freedom of motion. Start with the left leg slightly in front of the other one.

Find a comfortable rhythm in your belly-breathing while gently rotating the left hip forward and backward, feeling for the angle that provides the most fluid action in the joint. Reverse the rotation. Repeat the action with the feet in a horizontal line, then with the left leg slightly behind. Switch sides and repeat.

Group 3: Sense, place, listen, breathe

Follow the guidance for Group 1 and include a space to listen for your body's response to each change in position, and for each series of rotations. Pause for a few seconds while the soft tissue reorganizes. There will likely be a reseating of the head of the femur in the hip socket, some softening of the back muscles, and even of the feet as the ankles unwind. Wait for the changes to complete before continuing. You can explore the rotations with more weight on the right leg to see if additional benefits arise, then switch sides.

Many of the activities that are normally done standing will become easier after using these movement sequences. Posture will most likely also improve without you having to hold yourself up in a specific posture using muscle power. By achieving greater balance between systems, and releasing forces on the midline, there will also be more energy available to go through the day with increased ease, comfort, efficiency, and relaxation. It's natural for the focus to shift to whatever's in front of you as you move through the day, but it's very helpful if you also bring part of your attention back to your body to see if the neutral baseline has been lost a bit, so you can return it before it gets way off.

If you find yourself tightening up after being at a desk or on the computer for long periods, it could be very useful to stand for a few minutes and use one of the sequences to take the strain off your system. Even borrowing a few moments from your lunch break to reset will make the rest of the day pass much more easily for your body. Before bed is also a great time if your day is too full to squeeze it in beforehand. It's also great to do them as soon as you wake up, so your body can undo the fascia shrinkage that happens at night. The next series will be done lying down while facing up.

Remember that whatever improves posture improves the flow of information and regulation of the system between the three brains, and also key in my opinion, is the fourth brain: the bones.

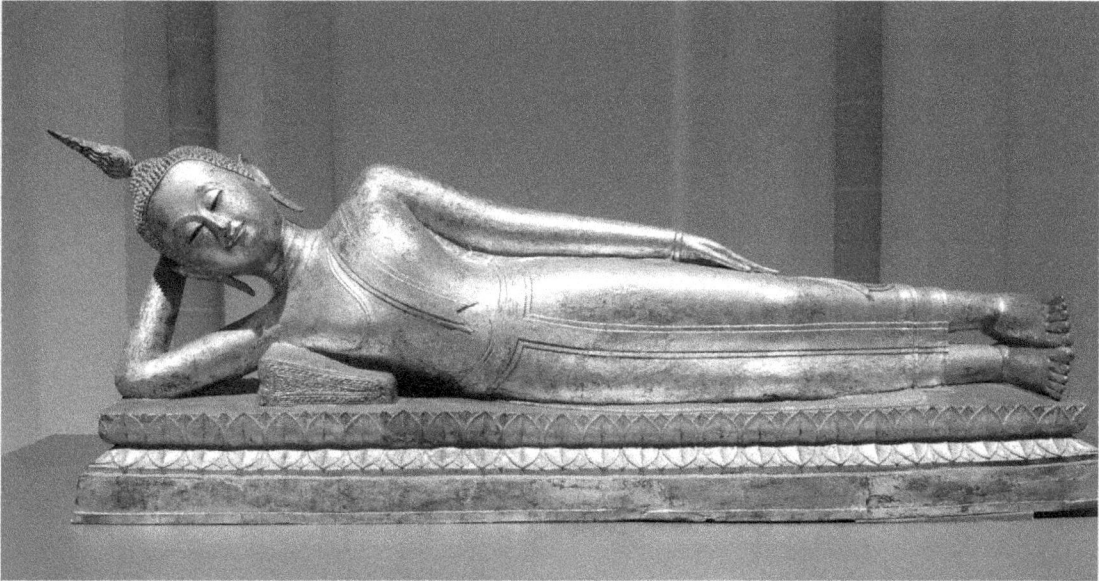

Section 4

Somatic Explorations While Supine
Manual Therapy for the Midline

❝ _____

An individual heals as distortions of influences from material and non-material sources resolve into symmetry

R. Paul Lee, D.O.
_____ ❞

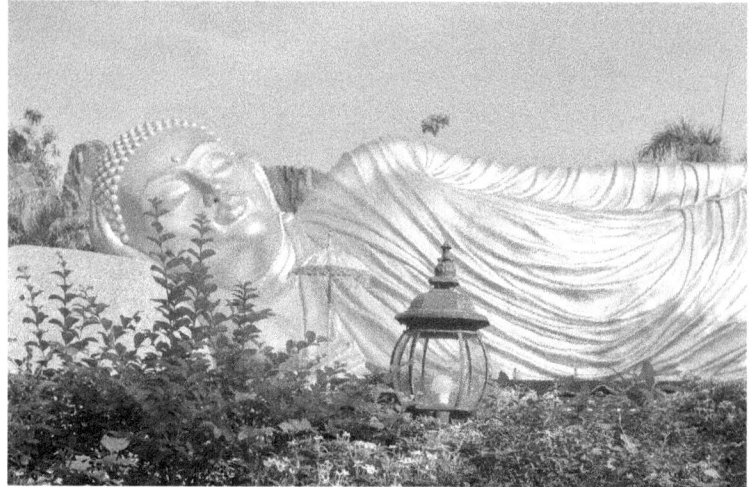

Chapter 5

Freeing the Midline through the Diaphragms

There are different gravitational and biomechanical forces that come into play while lying down. Sleep positions may have habituated certain patterns into your system, particularly if you're a side-sleeper or sleep on your belly at night. Keep those positions and patterns in mind as you relax on your back and do a brief scan for where your body may feel more dull, heavy, thick, or tense, and could use some re-awakening and resetting. See if what you notice in this position differs from what was revealed while standing. Cats and dogs often stretch their spines after lying down just for this purpose we assume, which also adds readiness for movement.

This position also adds support for your body while we explore combination sequences that would be awkward or strenuous while standing. It's best to send and receive information throughout the system while it's open and relaxed rather than challenging and straining the system to garner more strength. While being focused and gentle, slow and specific, there will be new layers of access that become available to your awareness, and to your body's ability to reveal those layers of activity. Big movements that require a lot of exertion have their own purpose. But this is similar to trying to hear the sound of a small fountain while standing in front of a waterfall. In this case, you're learning to hear the sound of your body connecting with itself, with you, and with its ability to return to balance. Being slow and gentle opens the "inner ears" that can hear the fountain.

Connecting the four main diaphragms

It was discussed in an earlier text how, in certain approaches to the body, there is more than one diaphragm. Various types of cranial sacral methods address these types of subdivisions in the body as diaphragms. There is one between the pelvic and abdominal cavities, between the abdominal and thoracic cavities (true respiratory diaphragm), between the thoracic and throat area (thoracic inlet) (Fig. 5.1), and between the throat and cranial cavities. They tend to be areas similar to major intersections where a significant amount of blood vessels and nerve fibers pass through, connecting sections of the body in a vital way.

They also potentially capture forces being transmitted from above or below due via the horizontal membranes that are often a characteristic of these diaphragms. If there is tension or malalignment in any of these areas, it could produce pressures in the areas above and below them, as well as having a significant effect on the vessels that must pass through the openings. Some have taken the position that the epiglottis at the back of the throat and the ethmoid/crista galli junction with the falx behind the bridge of the nose are also diaphragms, as well as the tentorium cerebelli at the back of the head. Anyone who's had a head injury can attest that manual therapy there is beneficial and balancing.

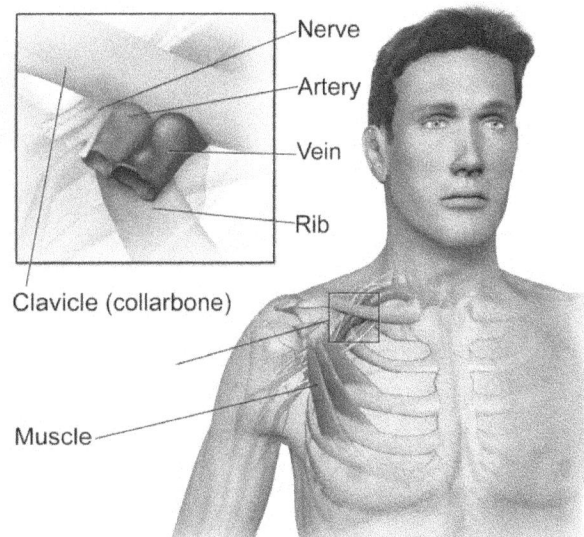

Fig. 5.1 – *Thoracic inlet/outlet area*, the center of which, at the top of the sternum, is considered to be one of the upper diaphragms
Courtesy of BruceBlaus, CC BY-SA 4.0 via Wikimedia Commons

As with the previous explorations with structures along the midline, pairing them by holding two areas simultaneously gives them a frame of reference with which to orient themselves in relationship to one another. It facilitates these sections reorganizing in a more balanced way, neutralizing existing tensions into a more coherent pattern. As tissue fields reorganize, restrictions in fluid flow and nerve transmission will be lessened. Whether or not you feel them come into balance between one another, or with other diaphragms, as with some of the other manual explorations, a noticeable calm will arise in the system as tensions abate.

ONE SKY

Diaphragm 1 – Cranial Connections

Group 1: Use soft hands and hold gently

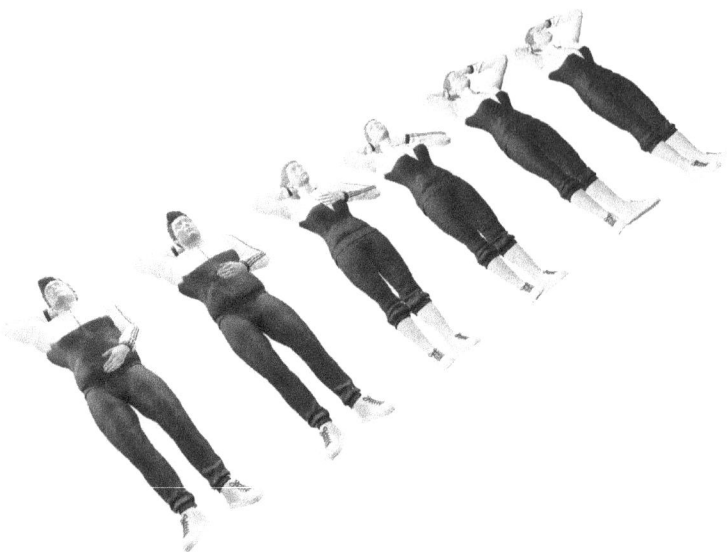

This hand position at the back of the head will be the stable hand that doesn't move. Although many structures are back there at the base of the cranium, your focus will be on the gentle, nurturing presence in your hands.

From there, place the other hand gently on the eyes first, with a focus on the ethmoid bone just behind the bridge of the nose. Then move that hand to the forehead, the thoracic inlet, the solar plexus, and the space between the ASIS of the pelvis. Hold each hand position for three belly breaths. Afterwards, bring the moving hand to your heart and hold it there for 3 breaths.

Group 2: Sense, breathe, and hold

Follow the general instructions for hand placement in Group 1, and within each location sense the space between your hands while maintaining awareness of any sensations throughout your whole body. Let your breath fill the space between your hands, and be mindful of the way your cranium, ribs, abdomen, and pelvic bowl move with your breath.

Notice what happens in your skin and joints with each breath. See if there is a separate, noticeable rhythm that becomes apparent aside from the pace and pattern of the breath.

Group 3: Sense, listen, breathe, and pause

Replicate the guidance from the other two groups, giving yourself time to listen to the body's responses. If there is any internal adjusting in response to the hand placement or breath, let it resolve before changing your hands.

Notice changes in the cranial base, including the bones and their felt sense of density or hardness, and whether you can feel some softening and opening of the diaphragms beneath your hands, any increased pulsations related to blood flow, or any relaxation happening in various areas of your spine and sacrum. Tune in to the current relationships between the diaphragms and how they make adjustments in response to one another.

ONE SKY

Exploring the diaphragms through the extremities and umbilicus

The extremities–arms, hands, legs, and feet–have an inescapable impact on the core. The core (or midline) attempts to stabilize and balance all of the forces, momentum, and actions initiated at the extremities. The limbs act as long levers for both engaging and releasing tensions in the core. The amount of weight and compressive forces added to the midline by whatever we carry with our arms is so great, that it's best to tuck it in tight right next to the chest or side to minimize those extra pounds of force. That includes what happens while we're doing the dishes, cooking, typing, washing the car, and so on. Accumulating forces is unavoidable, so it's very helpful to have something in your resource belt to unwind them all the way up the chain, from one end of your body to the other.

Diaphragm 2 - Freeing forces on the thoracic inlet

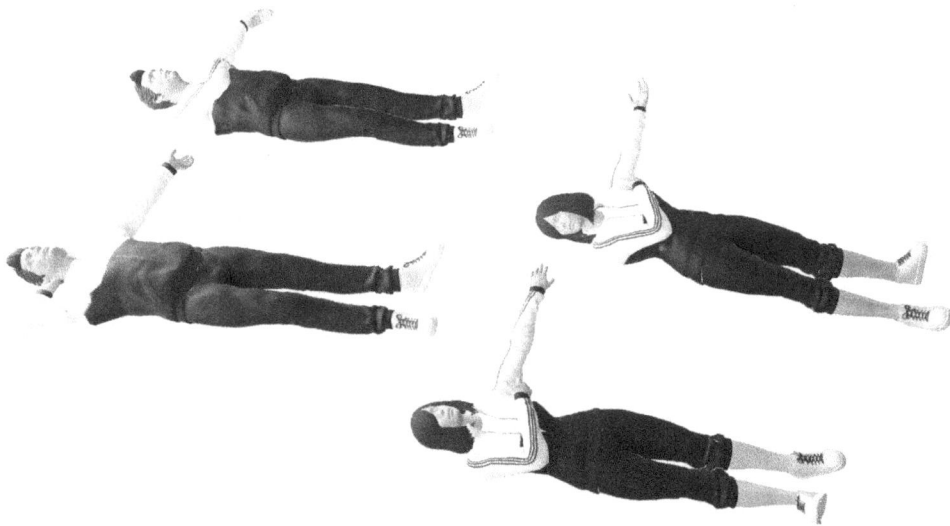

Upper diaphragms

During this sequence, your hand will have a soft, yet firm grip on the tissue between the ribs and the upper part of your arm–mostly the pectoralis muscles. This is right in the region of the thoracic inlet and where there's a considerable amount of blood and lymph flow, along with points for some of the meridians in the arm. You will be gently pulling the tissue toward your ribs and holding it there while the arm and shoulder (girdle and joint) are slowly extended and retracted, or decompressed, and slightly compressed. As you tune in more frequently, there will be additional sensations and responses that reveal themselves as your system continues to awaken and open. The changes, along with your awareness, will become more nuanced.

Group 1: Hold, move toward and away

While your right hand is cradling the back of your head, bring the left arm to shoulder height with the palm facing up toward the ceiling. Gently pull the arm in toward the shoulder socket, then reach away, extending the arm out of the socket just a bit.

After repeating this action 2 or 3 times, use the hand that was behind your head to gently grasp the muscles in front of the armpit of the outstretched arm, as if you were holding the scruff of a kitten's neck. Maintain the position of the tissue in front of the armpit with your grip as you slide the arm away, then back toward the socket.

The next time you pull the arm in toward the shoulder, also slide the hip on the left side up in the direction of your waist. Turn your head toward the right shoulder. Extend the arm out and away from the shoulder socket, and reach out and away from the hip with your leg and foot.

Bring your foot up (dorsiflex) in the direction of your shin at the same time, and gently turn your head in the opposite direction without straining.

Let each movement be slow and gentle. Let your palm face down toward the floor, then down toward your feet on alternating retractions and extensions of the arm and leg. Then switch sides.

Group 2: Move, sense, and breathe

Follow the general instructions for Group 1, but take a moment with each hand placement to inhale deeply and notice where the skin and tissue expand. Do you feel it at the base of your skull, do your ears move, your collar bones, or pelvis? Does the breath change the shape or position of your thighs, forearms, or feet?

When you clasp the pectoral muscles, what changes down the arm or in the thorax? What happens in your neck when you extend the arm away? Does it change more when you inhale or when you exhale?

Does your body prefer to inhale, move, and then exhale; or inhale, exhale, and then move? Which position of the palm allows more release to happen in the shoulder or neck? Can you sense the influence of the position of your hip on the neck and shoulder?

Explore holding the extended reach positions with the arm and leg while you take 3 belly breaths. Does your body release more with the head rotated toward or away from the left side? Compare how the other side feels when you switch, and see whether the right side has the same preferences for release as the left side.

Group 3: Move, breathe, pause, sense

Replicate the directions for Groups 1 and 2, but allow time at the outset of each new position to listen to any sensations that arise in your body. Where do the sensations arise when the right hand is behind the cranial base?

Allow a moment for your body to respond. Do you notice a type of 'echo' in the respiratory and pelvic diaphragms when you inhale? What happens in the other diaphragms when you extend and retract your arm? Can you feel the connection through the upper traps into the cranial base as the arm position changes? After a few repetitions, do you notice more freedom between the neck, arm, and shoulder in a way that achieves less pulling down through the fascia and vessels? Where do you feel a response with the neck rotations and leg extensions? Are you able to notice more freedom and less tension after combining your breath with the varied sequences?

Make a mental note of which areas feel the most easily and fluidly engaged with the movements, and which areas may feel a little clumsy or not fully integrated. Add repetitions for the clumsy areas.

Lower diaphragms

During this series, we'll use the umbilicus (the navel) as a point of organization around which the limbs can relate to one another as well as the core. There is so much packed into the midline and the center of gravity in the abdominal cavity, that it's easy for things to become restricted in nearby muscles or organs. Many people have had surgeries in the navel or groin area, making the area even more complex in terms of force vectors. It would already be complex due to the way each person's gait patterns have transmitted forces up the chain, so we'll be incorporating several different angles and combinations of sequences in order to account for these entanglements.

Diaphragm 3 - Lower diaphragms : respiratory and pelvic diaphragms

(Image examples provided may not be in the order of the sequence in descriptions)

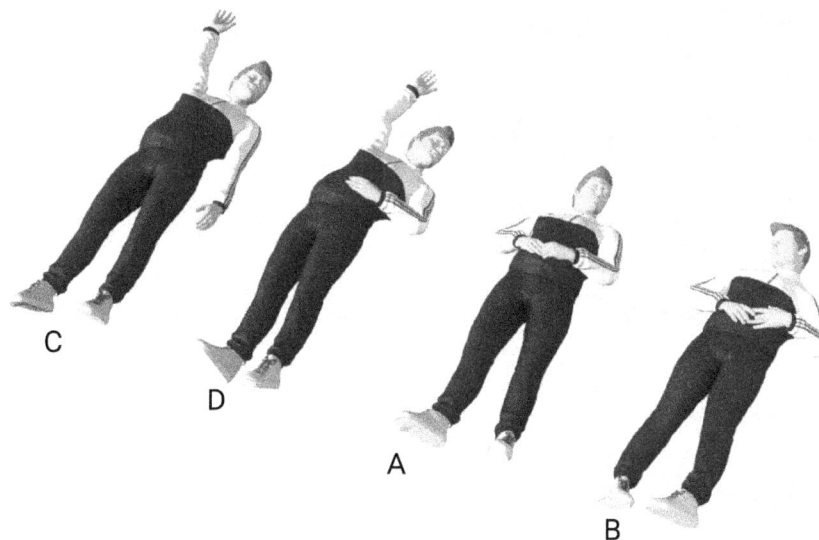

A - Place two fingers in the navel and pull up gently toward the same side shoulder as the extended leg, with toes pointed.

B - While your fingers are in your navel, pull up gently toward the left shoulder as you internally and externally rotate your legs and feet.

C - Reach up with one arm and down with that same leg, changing the position of the hand and foot on that side.

D - Reach up with one arm and down with that same leg while alternating moving the navel in the direction of the outstretched arm, or the extended leg

111

ONE SKY

Group 1: Go slowly and gradually within each movement without reaching for the end range

1. Don't use the navel if you have a hernia or mesh. Begin by placing your two middle or index fingers just a bit inside your navel. Gently **pull up** with your fingers as you **reach away** with one foot, toes pointed (A). **Retract that hip**, then reach again with the leg while you gently **pull down** on the navel. **Retract** the hip, **pull the navel up at an angle** toward the right shoulder, then **reach away** with the right heel. Retract the left hip and reach away with the left heel, leaving the navel where it is.

2. Repeat while pulling the navel gently up toward the left shoulder. Combine these movements with the legs and navel with a rotation and elevation (extension) of the head and neck. Then **combine these movements** with the **feet** turned outward and inward (B). Explore these combinations with a gentle **arch and curl** of your lower back.

3. Then reach up with one arm, extending out of the shoulder as you pull down just a bit with the navel, and reach away with one foot on the same side, then the opposite side (D).

4. Then reach up with one arm without the finger in the navel as you experiment with different positions of the feet as you reach with one hip, and then the other (C). Does it feel freer?

Group 2: Sense, breathe, and move gradually

1. Explore the suggestions for Group 1 while sensing the influence of each breath upon the abdominal cavity. Does the navel experience more restriction in relation to the movement of the hip and leg, or of the arm? Sense the differences in sensation between the right and left sides, as well as between the upper and lower diaphragms.

2. What happens in the respiratory diaphragm as you rotate the legs internally and externally? Notice which place in the leg rotation exerts the most or the least amount of tension coming through the navel and onto the diaphragm. After you discover the position of the most ease in the rotation, add the extension of the hip and leg away from the navel. Breathe deeply right there and notice if more space opens up.

3. Repeat this process using internal rotation of the arm and hand. Which shoulder and wrist accept the movement more readily? Does the arm with the most tension in the hand also have the most tension in the elbow or shoulder? How does the diaphragm on that side feel? Find the most neutral position for all of the joints in the rotation before extending the arm again, and check the diaphragm again.

4. Then use this neutral position of the arm in combination with varied angles of pull upward on the navel: toward the right or left shoulder, toward the chin, toward the lateral edge of the neck on either side, and toward the 9th rib on each side, and so on.

5. Use the same method to find the most neutral position for the feet. Explore these angles again with the navel while the feet are rotated internally and externally. Be aware of how each leg position and reaching away feels in the pelvic bowl and pelvic diaphragm (the space between the ASIS on both sides.) The goal is to discover equilibrium between various positions of the extremities right through the umbilicus and the diaphragms.

6. Once you've found the greatest amount of ease in reaching through the navel and diaphragms using the arms and legs, add the extension and flexion of your head and neck with small amounts of rotation. Continue to vary the combinations of rotation, reach/retraction, extension and flexion with your breath until you feel you've achieved freedom where there used to be tension and resistance.

7. Remember which diaphragm presented with the most tension initially, then add the combination of reaching with the arm and the leg while you're simultaneously varying the positions of the head and neck.

Group 3: Sense, breathe, pause, listen, and move

1. Replicate the guidance for Groups 1 and 2 while adding a pause to wait for the slow-moving viscera to adjust itself as you move the navel into new positions. Notice if there are any sticky places in the groin or pelvic bowl as you initiate a reach with the hip and leg, or an opposing pull with the navel.

2. Take a deep belly breath and hold it for a few seconds as you become aware of the areas that filled out and expanded with your breath. Wait a couple more seconds to allow for the tissue field to adjust itself before your exhale. Then hold the exhale and pause to allow the tissues to change again around the organs, viscera, and groin.

3. Compare which side receives the breath the easiest, and notice when it equalizes. Explore using a downward pull with the navel to follow the movement of the legs if both sides feel stiff or resistant. Find the most neutral position with the feet with rotation internally or externally, and pause to allow the tissue and other joints to respond.

4. Focus on the respiratory diaphragm as you inhale again, and notice which side feels the most elastic and receptive. Pull up with the navel toward the looser side as you reach with the opposite leg away from the navel. Exhale fully and hold it to see if you gain a bit more reach with the leg.

5. Inhale again and slowly rotate the foot until you feel a response/connection up through the leg and into the diaphragm. Hold that position and exhale, pausing for any additional global releases that may come. Revisit the internal or external rotation with the leg and foot, and check whether they now have a greater reach; a clearer transmission of elasticity all the way up the chain to the diaphragm or navel.

6. Repeat this sequence with different positions of the leg, then add the arms one at a time. Experiment with pulling the navel up toward or away from the arm, and notice which option affords the most release between the arm and the foot. Try the same concept with arm rotations.

Exploring wrist and hand positions on the whole body

Tap Dance

Our hands are involved in practically everything we do throughout the day. They are combined with and wired into other areas of the body continually in one way or another, from one end to the other. Many areas of the body will relax when the hands are more relaxed and opened. We almost always use them in a position that has them facing down, so the muscles that lift the wrists and fingers and rotate the hands are often at play during the task at hand. Both ends of the arm impact the upper and lower diaphragms.

As with the feet and ankles, it's also helpful to employ the full range that is possible for the hand and wrist articulations in order for the related muscles to be able to fully lengthen and release cumulative tensions. We can, with the proper shoes and gait pattern, accomplish this more easily with the feet and ankles than we can with the hands. This may be why they have more of a tendency toward arthritic changes in the fingers as time goes by. This next sequence will facilitate the unwinding and release of shared use patterns in the hands, wrists, feet, and ankles right through the core and through all of the diaphragms.

*This movement may not work for you if you have a torn rotator cuff or frozen shoulder.

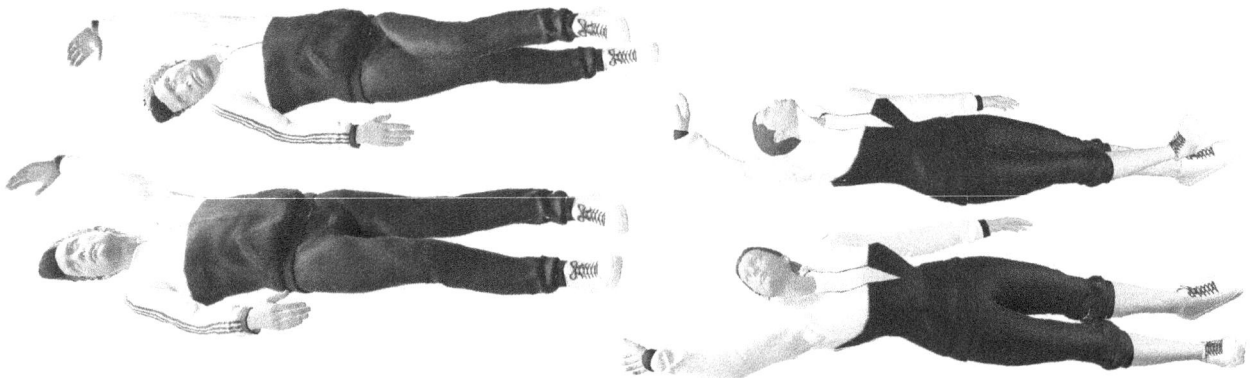

Group 1: Move into position gradually without strain

Start by changing the hand position of the arm that's above your head. Turn it around so the palm is facing upward with the back of your hand facing the top of your head. Gently move the arm closer to your ear if it's easy to do so. Then reach with the heel of that same side away from your center, having the leg externally rotated. Hold that position for 3 counts and turn your head to the opposite side. Try it with both an arched and a flat back.

Next, gradually bring the outstretched leg across the other one, exaggerating the lengthening of that side from fingers to toes. Extend your head and neck (chin up) and hold for three counts. Repeat on the other side. Then flip your hand around so the palm of your hand faces the top of your head with the chin down, and the head rotated to the other side. Reach with the leg and hip on that side, but have the toes pointed and leg internally rotated. Repeat on the other side.

Group 2: Inhale, sense the positions of ease, move, and exhale

Follow the recommendations for Group 1, but inhale before assuming the first position and feel where the sensations are the most prominent throughout the lower and upper arm as well as in the wrist and elbow joints. Slowly rotate your wrist until you find the most ease or least amount of tension, then exhale. There will often be a letting go with the exhale whereby you can move the arm further up nearer to your head with the elbow straighter. If this happens, take a deep breath before changing position, hold a couple of seconds, and do the same with the outstretched leg, which may also be able to reach farther. Switch sides and repeat.

Inhale and flip the hand into wrist flexion (facing down toward the head) as you internally rotate the hip and pivot the foot in the same direction. Exhale when you reach a comfortable end range, take up the slack of the softened tissues and reach a bit further with the arm and leg. Make small adjustments to the hand and foot positions to find another line of tension that doesn't strain the joints. Inhale and repeat the sequence.

Lift the outstretched leg slightly and cross it part-way over the other leg as you inhale and sense the areas in the IT band, ribs, and hip that may feel an extra lengthening. Exhale as you turn your head away a bit more, then inhale and replace the leg to the surface you're lying on. Compare the sensations and feedback from each side. If there's an area that calls out to you that still feels a bit restricted, see if you can access it using the hand and foot/leg positions we just went over, then reach away at different angles until you've contacted the exact place that didn't participate as fully beforehand. Pull into and reach out of that place a few times as you feel it expand and shrink with your breath, then relax in neutral and let everything settle.

Group 3: Inhale, sense the body's feedback, give time for its completion, and exhale

Follow the promptings for Groups 1 and 2, allowing time during the in and out breath to listen and wait for the tissue fields to reorganize. Rotate the arm, hand, and wrist intentionally to uncover areas of resistance and stop when you sense a barrier in the arm. Rotate the wrist to increase the tension slightly then inhale and reach.

Change the angle of internal or external rotation in the leg and amount of dorsiflexion versus plantarflexion in the foot until it increases the felt sense of resistance along the side of the leg or thorax. Once you find it, take a deep breath, include the head and neck in the pattern, allow the space to respond and reorganize, then exhale and repeat the sequence. Switch sides and make note of any differences you notice in each position between the right and left sides.

Freeing the arm and hand from the deltoids

This movement may help your entire side. Fascial chains along the side are structurally and functionally intertwined into patterns so that they all need to be addressed for any area to fully let go. If you're a rock climber, carry a briefcase, golf, work at a computer or cash register, play an instrument, use sciccors or use tools repetitively, you probably have residual tension along your arm. If so, the following exploration for the deltoid muscles (Fig. 4.8) should help.

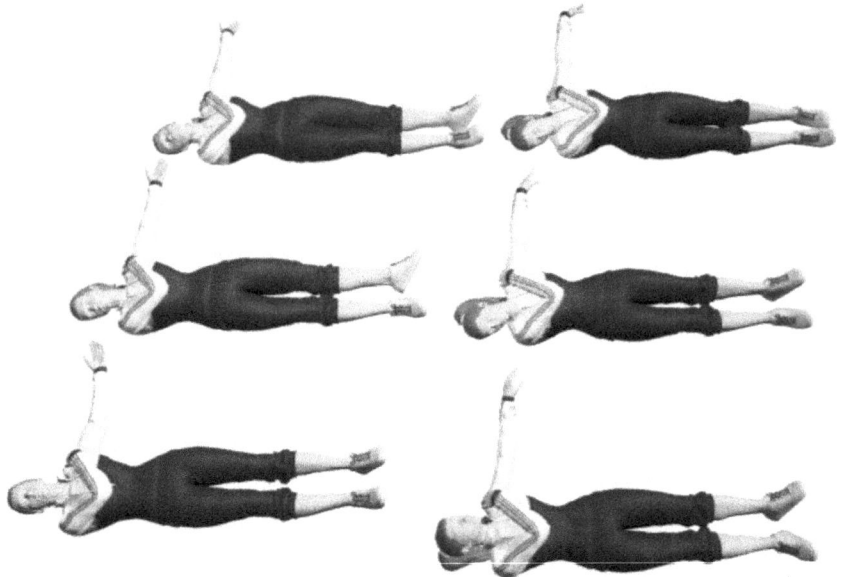

Tootsie Roll

Group 1: Use a firm but gentle grasp, reach and rotate

Cup as much as you can of the anterior, middle, and posterior deltoid muscles as you slide them toward the very top of your shoulder joint. Secure them at the highest point without forcing, and reach out and away from your shoulder socket with the arm.

Release your grip to change the position of your hand, wrist, fingers, head, and neck as you find new lines of tension. Then secure the grip again and gently, slowly rotate the arm while you maintain your grasp. Repeat the sequence while pushing the deltoids down toward the elbow. Change sides and follow the same procedure, without straining or squeezing too hard.

Group 2: Hold, sense, breathe, and move

Replicate the instructions for Group 1, but add the inhale as soon as you place your hand on the deltoids. Notice how the arm and shoulder expand with the breath, then pull the muscles up and sense whether the tissue fields relax more with the inhale or the exhale.

Which part of the arm produces the most sensation, either of tightening or releasing as you rotate the arm and change hand positions? Which direction of rotation is the easiest for your arm? Adjust how much you extend out of the socket and notice which place is the most effective for opening and softening.

Group 3: Use breath and position as fulcrums as you sense the body's feedback

Use the directions for Groups 1 and 2 for this group, and pause after placing your hand on the deltoids and taking a breath. Wait to see if the body is already starting to unwind all the soft tissue fields connected to the deltoids along with the deltoids themselves. Do the same for both the inbreath and the outbreath and notice which one affords the most release. Explore inhaling more into your sides versus your belly or chest and make note of the effects on the arm and shoulder.

Take your time with each change of position of the hand and wrist to sense where the lines of tension fall, what your breath does to influence the paths of unwinding, and whether it varies in your dominant versus non-dominant hand. Take time to notice which angle of the wrist and hand, and which position in the rotation of the arm facilitate the most release. Pause there for a few seconds. Play with the combinations of flexion or extension of the wrist, and with having the fingers spread a little versus a lot, registering the sensations throughout the arm that are produced with each modification. Refer back to Figs. 4.5. and 4.7 to see what you're unwinding.

Explore lowering the height of your arm just an inch or so and proceed through the sequences. Does your arm release with more ease in the lowered position? Do the deltoids? Play with flattening and arching your back, noticing the influence those difference spinal placements have on the shoulder joint. Is the influence more or less depending upon the rotation of the arm or the position of the hand? Remember that the lats insert right there at the upper medial aspect of the humerus, so this sequence can also help your back.

Getting to know the ins and outs of these lines of force on the areas that collect tension during daily activities will help immensely in your ability to release them at the end of the day or when the accumulation begins to produce discomfort. It's possible and even helpful to view the body according to systems of organization, and to use each one as a fulcrum for your focus and intention, as well as for your body's point of reference. We generally think of joint mobility and muscle lengthening when we use movement as an architect of change, strength, and balance for the system. Our frame of reference then becomes range of motion, ease of motion, comfort (minimal pain or stiffness), and capacity for support.

Within somatic reeducation, we also want to include the perspective of how alert and responsive the cells can be, how much of the tissue field can open and attend to new information, and how efficient the communication is between systems. We look at fluidity, lucidity, dexterity, and integration as landmarks for the direction we want to embody, and as fulcrums for where we're leading the body's capacities. We've incorporated governors of the parasympathetic nervous and endocrine systems as fulcrums, the organs, diaphragms, posture, joints, extremities, skin, and lines of force as fulcrums that all affect the midline- the major conduit for communication that resets the system.

The next section will describe movements that are less common. They use positions that we don't often use in daily life, so they have the potential to create greater attentiveness in the brain. They can also challenge muscle memory to invite new options into its sphere that lead to increased interconnections and grace; that improve the quality and capacity of movement. It's like expanding your body's vocabulary.

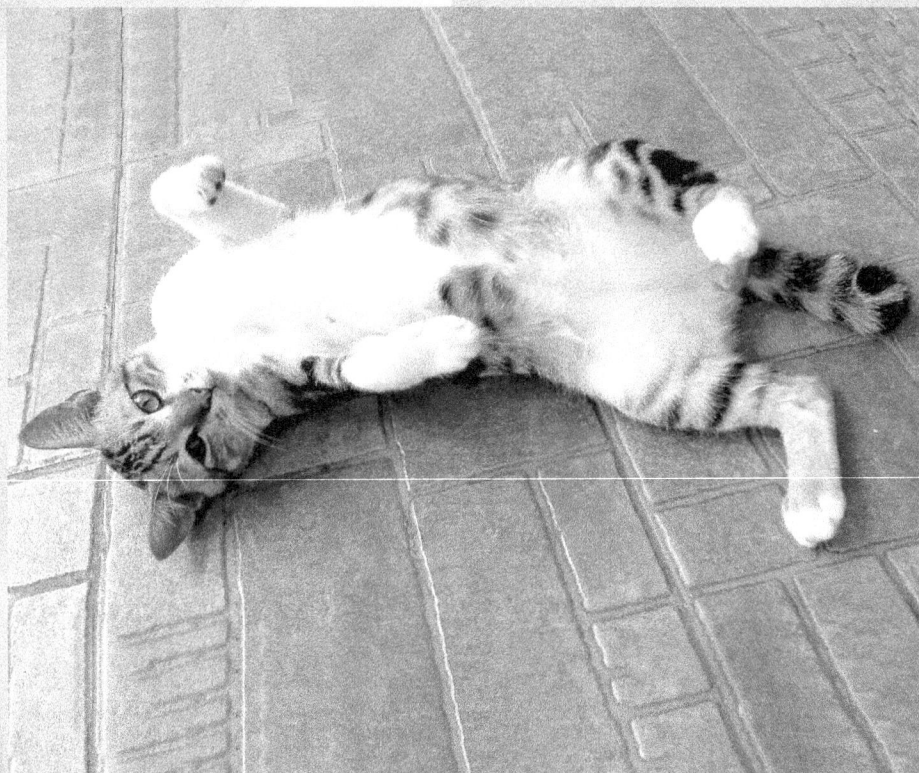

Section 5

Freeing the Midline from the Limbs

Side-Lying Somatics

Chapter 6
Freeing the Midline Using the Whole Body

Now that we've released a great deal of kinks, restrictions and various types of tension that may have been wired into the midline, we can explore bigger movements more freely. Little yummy, appreciative sensations may have already begun expressing themselves as dormant energies, and connections have begun to emerge all the way to the surface of your skin. As you've seen throughout the earlier explorations, there is no separation between the anatomy and physiology, (between structure and function). The nerve and blood vessels interpenetrate the bones and soft tissue, the lymph and meridians wrap around the blood and nerve fibers, and the cerebral spinal fluid pours into the lymph and blood vessels. The emotions, thoughts, hormones, neurotransmitters, nutrients, enzymes and bacteria circulate with the organs, glands, and many of the other systems listed above.

When we move, all of the above is also moving; is also being influenced by what and how we move, and by how we make contact with what moves. We are able to create and enjoy serenity and harmony through movement, as well as the bliss of millions of molecules that are able to function more effortlessly throughout your system. That sensation of contentment is your body's way of letting you know that you've come home. Bring that deepening relationship with your body into the whole-body movements we'll do now.

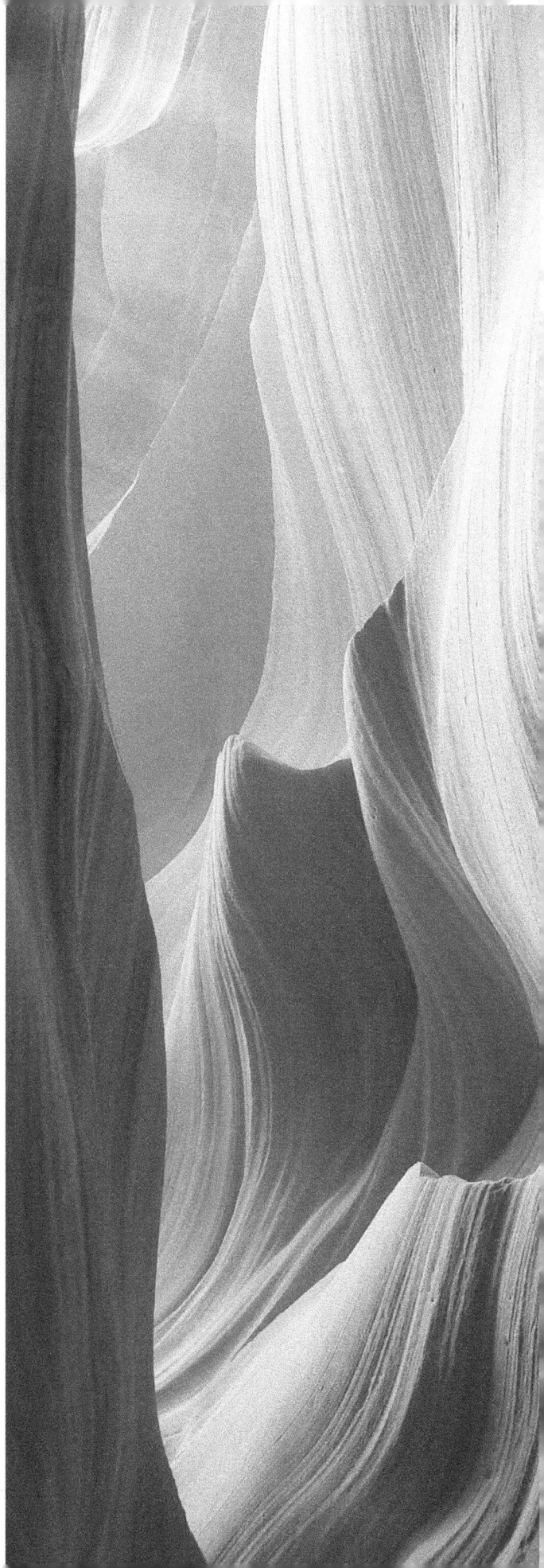

ONE SKY

Trees in the wind - moving forces freely through the core

The focus of these movements will be to consciously move everything in your body in a way which honors the recognition that everything in the middle, or midline, is responding is responding to each action at the furthest points. We've experienced and will explore further how the hands and feet can lead and influence the movement in ways that complement and coordinate the well-being of the core.

Now let's see how to make the movements smooth, effortless, graceful, and elegant. Find those angles and use of the breath that your body enjoys the most for each sequence. Have fun with them, and allow them to spark increased flows of energy in new ways that deepen the connections that have already happened within. Be aware of how they expand the relationship and understanding you've been developing with every part of your system.

For these next sequences, let your body move in its own way now that you've learned what it prefers and where it has the most ease. It's more about moving freely than about trying to do something correctly according to a roadmap toward a destination. It's all about the journey and enjoying the "scenery" along the way. Maintain awareness in the midline as you move, and take care that it remains as comfortable and relaxed, yet supportive as possible when the extremities are active.

Trees in the wind 1

Trees 1: All Groups Get comfy and move freely

Lie on your side on a surface that is firm but yields enough to make it easy on your hips and shoulders. Have the fingers of your upper arm point straight up to the ceiling while the arm is shoulder height, if possible. Lift the head of the humerus (arm bone) up and away from the socket like we did in an earlier sequence. Allow it to drift down using the pull of gravity, controlling a smooth, vertical descent back into the socket. **Inhale and lift, exhale and release back down**. Repeat a few times then lift the arm again, gradually allowing it to fall back behind you as you extend the wrist and lean your head in the opposite direction. You can also reach with your knee away from the shoulder to feel additional lengthening through the waist, ribs, and hip. Repeat a few times and change sides.

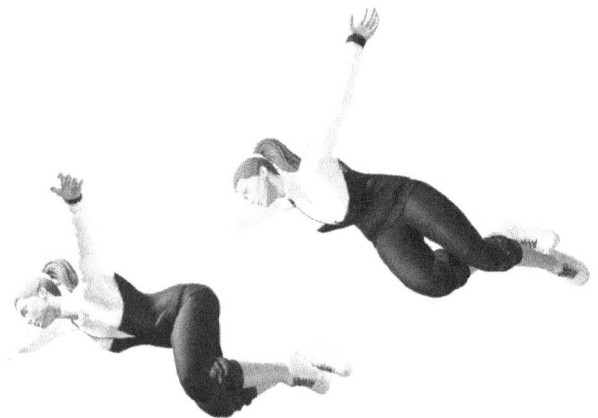

Trees in the wind 2

Let the arm swing backward and forward, then combine the forward arm with a backward leg, and vice versa.

Trees 2: Group 1 Move with ease

Repeat the guidance for Trees 1 and bring Make sure your arm, head, and neck positions feel comfortable before you begin the movement. Take your time, lift the arm, and maintain the most neutral position possible as you gently swing the arm forward and back. Let it be slow, smooth, and effortless.

Once you're comfortable with the arm and shoulder movement, add the hip and leg swinging smoothly (don't lift it, but slide it) in the opposite direction. Repeat a few times, then switch sides.

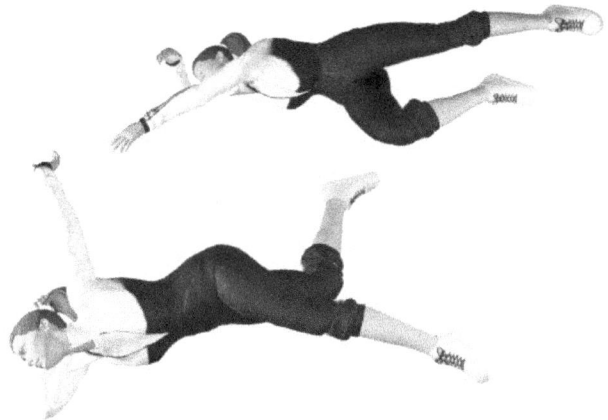

Trees 2: Groups 2 and 3 Breathe, sense, adjust, and move

Replicate the suggestions for Group 1 in general. After positioning yourself, sense the area around and inside the shoulder girdle and joint to find the best, most neutral placement of your arm. Take a deep belly breath and, with as much ease and fluidity as possible, lift your arm from the glenohumoral joint first, then reach toward the ceiling with your fingers.

Notice how smoothly it moves and if it wobbles, where in the upward motion it happens. Rotate the arm or hand slightly in each direction and see if it feels easier. Which muscles do you feel in your back, chest, and thorax as you reach away, and where do you feel sensation as it descends back into the joint. What happens in your ribs, organs, sides and hips when you extend the arm and shoulder in each direction?

Add the swinging of your leg into the motion and see if you can make it one continuous action-smooth and effortless along the entire route. Inhale with the lift, and exhale with the descent. Is there any modification you can make to your arm or shoulder that brings more ease to the leg and hip, or vice versa? Switch sides and make note of any differences as you sense one side in comparison to the other. Adjust the angle or rotation of your arm, your head and neck, pelvis, or legs to achieve as much ease and flow as possible for each, then for all of them together.

Trees in the wind 3 - Variations

Explore these slight variations in arm and hand placements and how they're combined with leg and foot positions. Focus on the ease and smoothness in the transitions. You want to experience integration from one end of your body to the other.

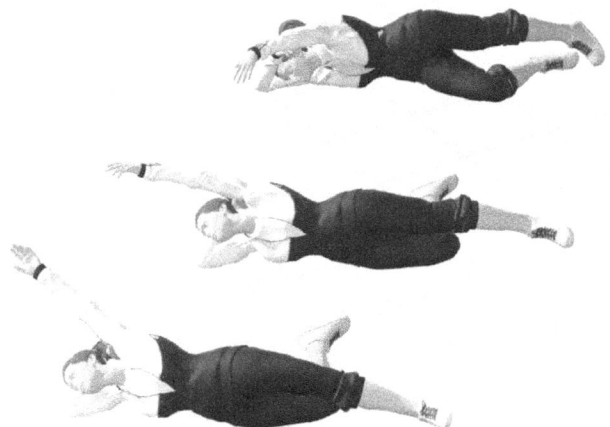

ONE SKY

All Groups : Sense, listen, pause, follow, and move

Experiment with what you've learned so far about what brings more ease and fluidity to a coordinated movement for your body. Search for any lines of tension in each position that may be either mutually limiting, or mutually liberating. Make the adjustments your body wants to make in the direction of more freedom or more comfort before and as you move. Apply what you've learned about using your breath.

Exhale while the arm is at its greatest extension, and sense what happens as the breath diminishes. Inhale again and notice if you now have more freedom. Extend your arm and wrist and slightly rotate your thorax and arm back as you reach away, then reach more forward with the thorax and arm. Experiment a bit with the placement of the upper leg.

Make the motion as smooth as though you were submerged in water, and keep the flow happening in every direction. Notice the natural tendencies for the lower body to move with the upper body, then do it with fluidity like an eel in the ocean. Change sides and check to see if the other side learned from the first side how to perform the sequence with ease.

Manual therapy for the hip and IT band

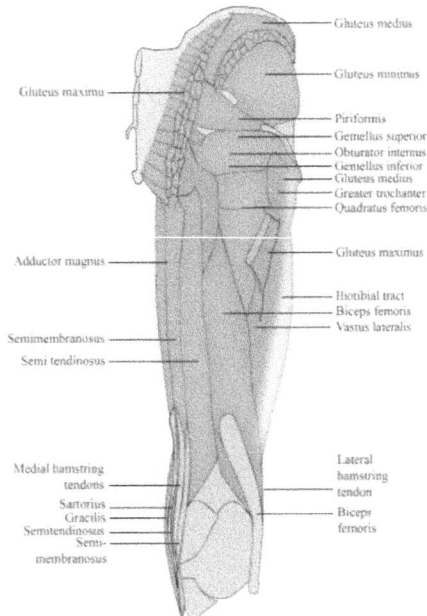

Fig. 6.3 – Muscles of the hip and thigh that can be helped by the next sequence

This area is a challenging one for many people who are active and athletic. There are a few muscles that attach to the greater trochanter that are small but pack a punch. The gluteus maximus, medius, and minimus get a hefty workout most days, along with the piriformis (Fig.6.2), which everyone who's had sciatica is most likely familiar with. The tensor fascia lata is a small muscle above the trochanter that morphs into the tendon that becomes one with the sheath we know as the iliotibial tract, or IT band.

Very often this tract becomes stiff due to compression in the knee joint or the peroneus muscle on the side of the lower leg, but we can also influence it from above. Being one of the bony prominences that tend to be a catch place for fascia, the greater trochanter is subject to many sources of potential tension or restriction (Fig. 6.1). This means that it can also be used as a fulcrum from which several different planes of action can be accessed and reset.

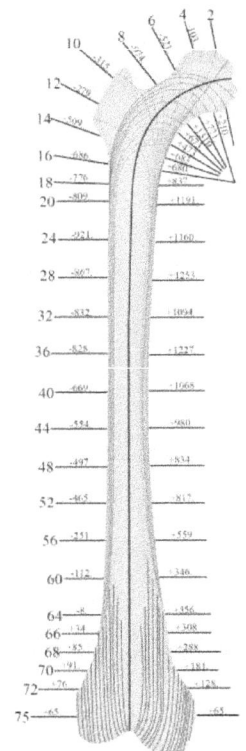

Fig. 6.1- Lines of stress along the femur and trochanter

Your **hand placement** for the next sequence will begin between the rim of the ilium and the greater trochanter, then proceed along the IT band toward the knee (Fig. 6.2).

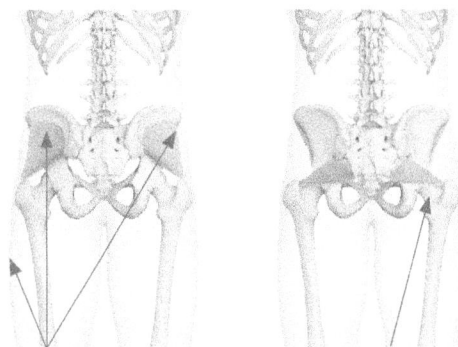

Fig. 6.2 - Gluteal and Piriformis muscles. Check Fig. 4.10 for detailed anatomy. Sense which layer may benefit the most from your contact and has the best affect on the IT band.

The Claw - Fascial reset for the lateral chain (hip and IT band)

Group 1: Grab, hold, reach, and retract

Lie on your side with comfortable support for your head and your hips. Have your knees bent at a 90° or 70° angle. Grab a hand full of flesh **just above the greater trochanter** (Fig. 6.2) and squeeze just enough so that the tissue barely moves when the leg moves. **Reach forward** slowly with your knee, and then pull back. Repeat a few times. If it burns, grab less tissue and just reach an inch or two; don't force it.

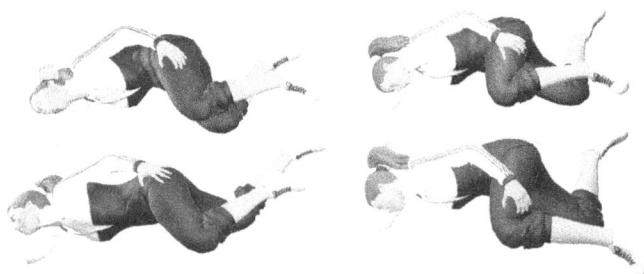

Reach down at an angle with your knee, and pull back again a few times, maintaining the firm grip of the flesh with your hand. Then place your hand **below the greater trochanter** and repeat the process. You may need to widen your grip and be more gentle, as this area can be tender. Gingerly work your way down the thigh to your knee, then switch sides.

Group 2: Hold, sense, breathe, and move

Follow the suggestions for Group 1, but take a breath when you find the best place to grab, and apply the amount of pressure that your body responds the best to. If the rest of your leg or body tightens, let go a bit and try a different or softer grip. Move the leg back and forth slowly, sensing the best angle for the most release in the hip and thigh. Notice whether the inhale works better with the extension or with the retraction. Maybe your body prefers to have the inhale and exhale both with the extension, then inhale and exhale again on the retraction. Find out.

When you move your hand below the trochanter, grab the lateral aspects of the quads and hamstring, then squeeze them together to sandwich the IT band. On the next pass, create a narrower grip so that you're just squeezing the IT band, and compare the effects. Experiment with your breath and hand placement as you work your way down the thigh. You can also try starting at the knee and working your way up the leg. Switch sides and repeat.

Group 3: Grasp, sense, listen, pause, breathe, and move

Repeat the instructions for Groups 1 and 2, but sense how your body responds to your grasp. Wait for the muscles to finish yielding and modifying before moving your hand. Take a breath and check in again to see whether there's more shifting in a wider area, or in a deeper layer. Hold the inbreath for a few seconds and pause for more unwinding of the tissue fields, then exhale and pause again. Compare the exploration of held breath with normal breathing as you move.

Experiment with changing your hand position to an angle, rather than a vertical line (as in 12 and 6 on a clock). Test a 1 and 7 o'clock angle, then try 11 and 5 to see how the tissue responds. Explore changing the angle of your leg also, modifying the horizontal plane of 3 or 4 o'clock with 5 or 6 o'clock as you reach away.

You can also vary the arm position for the inactive/passive side. There will be a very different organization of the tissue matrix if the arm is outstretched compared with it being bent under your head. Since there is a contralateral relationship between the right hip and the left arm and vice versa, there could be additional benefit to connecting them a bit more by changing position of the arm and feeling the link through the thorax and abdomen. Then switch sides.

Sequence for internal and external rotation of proximal joints

The rotator cuff (Fig. 6.4) is often vulnerable to injury in both males and females whether it be from sports, falls, or repetitive strain. They, like the hip rotators, are small but mighty. They work very hard for their size and endure quite a bit of force directly through the arms, and while paired with the hips and legs. These muscles are not so easy to touch with your hands but can be accessed using movement. In both cases, part of what we want to do for healthy maintenance, is to touch base with the muscles from time to time to awaken them and gently run through their functions to reclaim ease, freedom, and range of motion. You can use a light weight if you want to make their location more obvious to the brain and to your own sensing radar, but it's not necessary for them to unwind. This next sequence helps to awaken and reset the rotator cuff

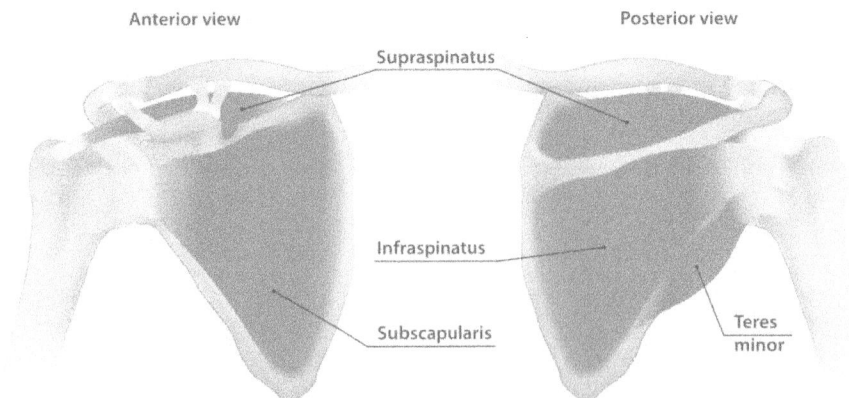

Fig. 6.4 – Rotator cuff muscles
Courtesy of InjuryMap, CC BY-SA 4.0 via Wikimedia Commons

The Happy Clam

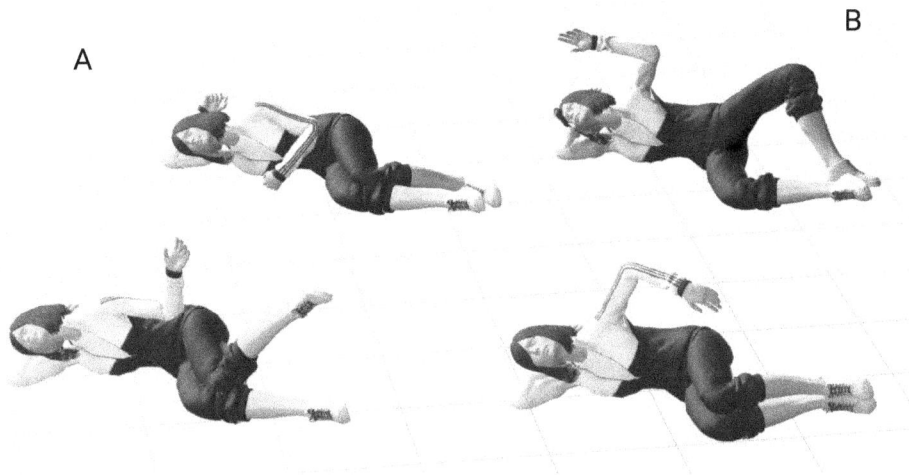

A

B

Group 1: Move slowly and in sync

You may want to skip this and the following sequences if you have a torn rotator cuff, adhesive capsulitis (frozen shoulder), or recent shoulder surgery. Find a comfortable place to lie on your side with support for your head. Have your upper arm resting flat on your side with your elbow bent at 90°. Your knees can also be bent at an angle between 70° and 90°.

From there, gradually rotate the forearm from its spot near your belly to being vertical with your fingers pointing to the ceiling. (A) At the same time, lift your lower leg while keeping your knees together. Then lower them gradually together to the count of 6.

Repeat 3 times, then make a comfortable 'L' shape again with your arm, this time having your upper arm straight out from the socket and vertical to the ground with the palm facing behind you while your forearm is parallel to your body (B).

Your knees will start out together, then lift the knee of the upper leg while keeping your feet together as you rotate/pivot your arm so that your forearm and palm face forward. Move them gradually in both directions a few times again, in sync, then switch sides and repeat the sequence.

Groups 2 and 3: Breathe, sense, and move as a harmonious unit

Replicate the recommendations for Group 1, and focus on the smooth slide and glide of the joints as they move together in harmony. Take fairly deep breaths before initiating a movement, and be sure that the head of the humerus is seated squarely in the glenohumeral joint before swiveling.

ONE SKY

You can also see how it feels to lift the arm out and away from the joint before swiveling. Experiment with breathing into your belly, into your chest, then into your sides, and then your back. Notice which respiratory focus affords the most ease in the action of the shoulder joint. Explore whether pausing at the peak of the inhale allows the upper traps or any other muscle group to let go more.

When lifting the lower leg, check whether or not the hip releases more if you allow the foot to go down past the other leg onto the surface you're lying on. For both actions of the leg, determine which angle gives the most release for the hip. Try switching it up so that the arm rotations of A are used with the hip rotations of B and vice versa. Be as fluid as you possibly can throughout the transitions in position.

The Rocking Chair

A – Move the shoulder with arch and curl   B - Move the hip, knee and neck

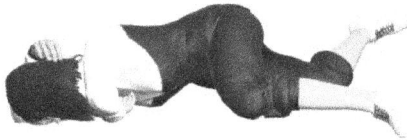

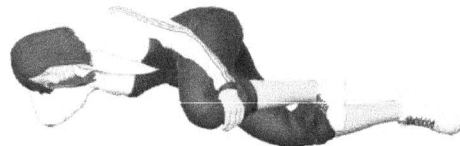

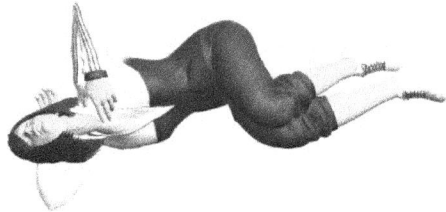

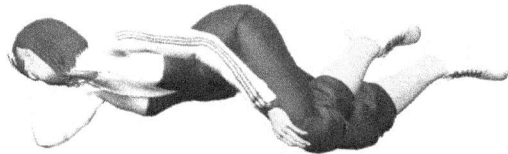

In this next sequence, the tone is one of a balmy early evening on the front porch in a warm breeze swaying back and forth in a rocking chair. We're still focusing on the proximal joints—the hips and shoulders—working in harmony together, letting the neck rock gently to and fro using the momentum of the other joints. Ease and comfort are premium aspects of the intention and direction of this exploration; just enjoying the sensation of moving freely. Lie on your back and relax for several seconds before switching sides.

Group 1: Find a rhythmic flow with each motion

Seek comfort in each position, allowing your torso to lead the motion and determine where your arms and legs wind up. Then, holding the knee of the top leg, gently pull it toward you as your head and neck roll in the direction that's most natural for your body, either toward or away from the knee (B).

Be as smooth as you can as you slowly rock back and forth in and out of this movement. Then change your hand position so that it's pushing the knee away from your head, and let the head and neck roll naturally again in sync with the leg.

Next, bring your arm up to shoulder height and bend the elbow, allowing the hand and forearm to remain relaxed. Reach forward with the elbow so that the shoulder blade also moves forward as you flatten your back. Then reach back with your elbow as you arch your back (A). Allow natural motion of your head and neck. Repeat a few times and switch sides.

Groups 2 and 3: Breathe, move, sense, and adjust

Repeat the suggestions for Group 1 as you add the breath into the flow of the movement. Check to see if motion is easier with the inbreath or the outbreath. Sense the position or angle of your knee so that the areas that benefit the most from the movement are being fully engaged.

For section A, feel the muscles of the shoulder girdle in the back as the scapula slides over your ribs, gently moving the rhomboids and lower traps. Feel what happens in your chest as the elbow glides behind you, and notice the sensation in between your shoulder blades as the elbow moves to the front.

How do the sensations change in your shoulder girdle and chest as you arch and curl your spine? Choose whether to allow your head and neck to move with your spine or with your shoulder. Notice if the smooth glide is the same on the other side.

Rocking and rolling the head and neck

As you can imagine, the neck gets quite a workout every day just holding up the head and negotiating its position in relation to the rest of the body on an ongoing basis. It also is unwittingly paired and wired into its relationship with the torso when we turn to look at something, and in relationship with the eyes as we drive, read, or text. It's best to differentiate these functions from time to time so that they don't become self-limiting. A little change in posture can have a strenuous impact upon the anterior cervicals (Fig.6.5), which in turn will put pressure on the upper trapezius muscles at the back of the neck.

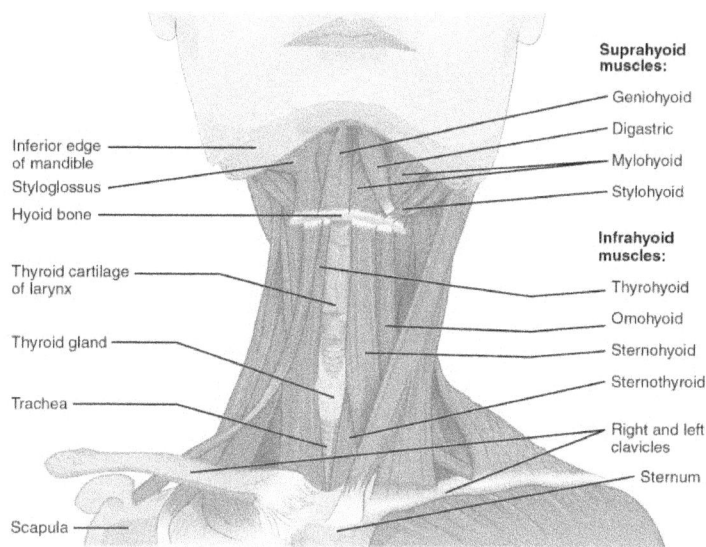

Fig. 6.5 - Muscles of the anterior neck
Courtesy of OpenStax, CC BY-SA 4.0, via Wikimedia Commons

The neck is a significant intersection for everything above and below it, so keeping the blood flow and nerve transmission clear and free in the neck and through the thoracic inlet can be very helpful. Since daily life, most occupations and hobbies will at some point strain the neck and shoulders, having a regular routine to release it is invaluable.

ONE SKY

Sitting and reading for prolonged periods or having a head-forward posture will put a strain on the sternocleidomastoid muscles, which are very strong, but that strength can also create discomfort. Since they not only lift, but also rotate the head, some movement that involves passive rotation of the head and neck will be able to release/inhibit tension in those muscles. If your head feels light instead of heavy during this next exercise, it means the muscles are participating rather than letting go into being passively turned. The supraspinatus tendon (Fig.6.6) is one that often becomes overworked, so take care that the position of the humerus in relation to the socket feels balanced and neutral.

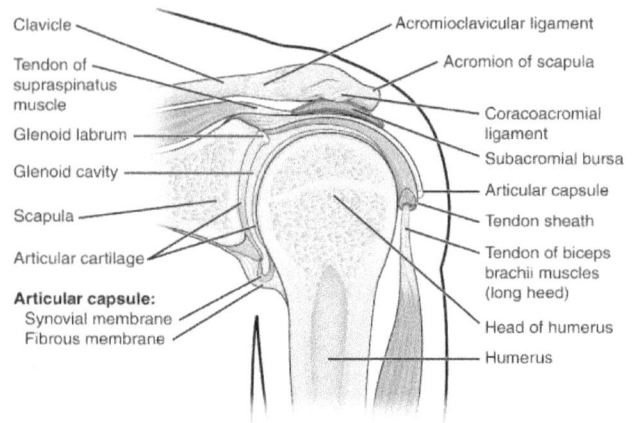

Fig. 6.6 – Shoulder joint anatomy
Courtesy of OpenStax College, CC BY SA 3.0, via Wikimedia Commons

The Rock and Roll

Group 1: Hold, lift, and lower

Skip this sequence if you have disc, spur, or major arthritic issues in your neck. Let your body be a single unit, like a piece of string on the water that rolls with the waves. Practice lifting your head gently with your hand without using your neck muscles. Only go as far as you can with your neck being relaxed.

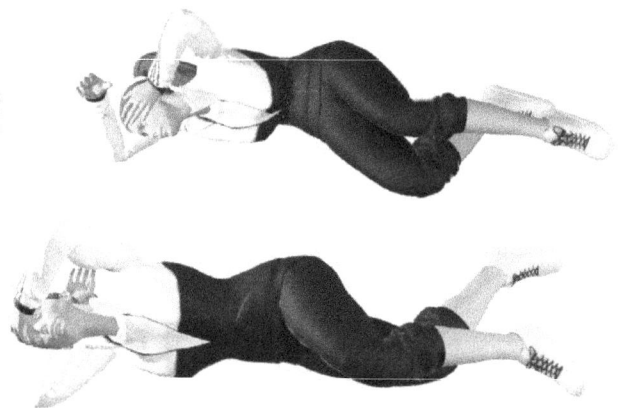

As you reach the peak of rotation toward the arm that's doing the lifting, place the hand on the other side of your head and softly press it back down. Don't press it straight down, but rather in a rotating, turning motion. Repeat the motion three times, then switch to the other side.

Group 2: Breathe, sense, lift, and lower

Follow the instructions for Group 1, and use your breath to help support and carry the motion effortlessly. Lift with the inhale and lower with the exhale, getting a sense of which angle of your head is easiest for a smooth movement. Notice if your chin should stay level, move up with the lift and down with the press, or something even more comfortable.

See if the best hand placement is on your forehead, by your cheekbone, in front of your ear, or vertical, where it pretty much covers the entire side of your face. Make the motion smooth and liquid, like you are rocking a baby in a cradle, but much slower.

Pay attention to the midline as you turn your head, and be aware of how far down the spine the motion goes. Do you feel the spine itself, or the soft tissue adjacent to the spine moving? Does the movement go farther depending upon hand position or the angle of your head? Make any adjustments that allow the motion to be more inclusive and more fluid.

Group 3: Sense, breathe, listen, adjust, and move

Lie down in the position that enables the most freedom of motion for your spine. Will your back be flatter, or more arched? Which placement of your hips and legs produce more tension in your spine, and which slight adjustment brings more neutrality and ease?

This sequence calls for smooth, graceful, whole-body motion, so make adjustments along the way that bring more ease. It doesn't always need to involve holding and waiting for the body to make adjustments. Listen to what the body reveals is the better way and position to move from, and even if it's just an inch, make those modifications. When your body feels safer, it will let go more.

It may change because things will be releasing and softening along the way, bringing more freedom and increased options. More and more areas will be able to find comfort in a wider range of positions. Notice which ways your breath can bring even more fluidity and ease to each movement, and more awakening in your spine. Notice when more awakening offers additional feedback as you move so you can continue to adjust.

The Neck Roll

For this sequence, care must be taken to gently hold the skin without squeezing it. The hand is placed securely so it won't slip, but stays in place on the surface of the skin as the head and neck rotate from side to side. The skin is a major communicator for the rest of the system on a cellular level. The contact is therefore not intended as a stretch or myofascial technique, but is using the skin and fascia to bring other layers up to date on their status, so move slowly. You will also be addressing aspects of the gut tube, so positive changes can happen throughout the thorax, abdomen, and pelvis.

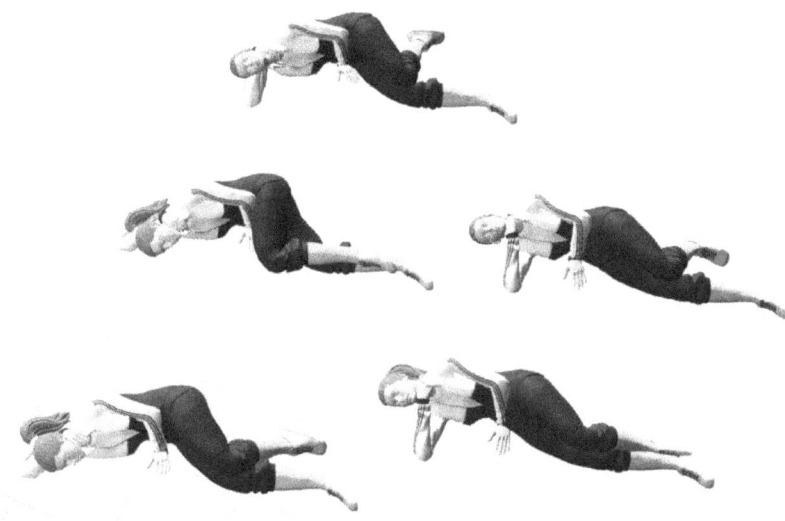

Group 1: Make gentle contact and gradually rotate the neck and head

Find a stable position on your side with support for your head and neck, and place your hand around your neck like a soft, snug scarf with fingers facing down toward the ground. Hold steady in that place on your neck and gradually rotate your neck in the opposite direction—toward the ceiling to the count of 10-then rotate your head down toward the ground, just as slowly. Gradually arch your back when your neck rotates up, and flatten it as your neck rotates down toward the ground.

Come around to the front of your neck, being careful to not place any pressure on your throat, esophagus, or any of the sensitive structures in your neck. Your fingers will still be facing down. If you feel your heartbeat, soften your grip until you don't feel it. Rotate your head up toward the ceiling gradually to the count of 10, then back down again to the count of 10. Relax on your back for a few seconds before you switch sides.

Group 2: Sense, breathe, adjust, move slowly

Follow the guidance for Group 1, and breathe into the motion as though the movement was floating on the breath. Inhale on the way up with your head, and exhale on the way down.

Find out if there is a different angle in the placement of your fingers that will allow more ease in the rotation and more release in your neck. Also monitor the angle of the side-lying position to see if a slight variation helps the head and neck let go more fully; to have more support.

Bring your knees closer, and then further from your chest while your hand is on your neck, and notice what happens. Find the placement of your legs that brings the most ease into your neck muscles. Do the same for the arch, flattening, or curl of your back. Which one affords the most relaxation for your neck?

After discovering the most neutral positions for the contributing influences on your neck, begin moving with the breath. Does your neck like to extend and lift the chin a bit while rotating up and flex the neck a bit while rotating downward? Or does it prefer to stay even? Continue to explore your systems preferences that bring the most ease, glide, and effortlessness as you move.

After 2 or 3 repetitions of each hand position, relax on your back for several seconds. Then switch sides and notice if the preferences are similar or different on the other side. When you've learned the preferences, explore making the breath, rotation, arching and curling of your back one smooth action, remaining gentle, gradual, and now global.

Group 3: Sense, breathe, pause, listen, adjust and move

Use the instructions for Groups 1 and 2, and add a pause after taking a breath to listen and wait for your body to respond to your touch. The upper lobe of the lung is very near the first rib, which is very near where your hand will be, so there will be changes in the tissue with the first breath.

The skin may begin to release right away and open to deeper layers, so take care not to let your hand drop with more weight in this process. Blood vessels like being stretched but may not receive direct pressure as well, so if you feel the pulse in the carotid artery, lighten your pressure.

The body responds even more to input combined with movement, so after the tissue resets with the inhale, begin to rotate your neck and notice the additional response in layers of the skin and muscles. Pause for it to do its own unwinding, and if it's time for the exhale, go ahead and let the breath go. Experiment with how much additional change will happen in the layers of your neck by including movement for your back. Try arching with the inbreath, and curling with the outbreath to see what may change throughout the thorax that can also open more unwinding in the neck, shoulders, and spine.

Then reverse the pattern and inhale as you flatten and curl your spine, and exhale with the arch, waiting for your system to respond to the new input. Add the potential extension and flexion of the neck if your body likes it, and move in harmony with all of the modifications. Let your body move as a fluid, conscious whole.

After freeing up areas in the upper diaphragms via the neck is a perfect time to revisit the cranium. It is supremely calming and integrating to hold the base of the skull and sacrum at the same time. Many subtle changes can occur during this hold that may or may not be too subtle to sense because some of what happens is through the nutritive factors in the fluid exchanges. The influence on the central nervous system will be much easier to feel because the relaxation that follows is unmistakable. The side-lying position is best for this contact with oneself, but you still need to find the most comfortable option for the hand and arm that will be behind your back.

Dr. Michael Kern states that, "In essence, the mid-tide is an expression of the embodied forces of the Breath of Life. The Biodynamic potency expressed within the mid-tide is of great significance because it carries into the body the essential ordering forces of the Breath of life. Therefore it has a profound ability to maintain physiological integration and balance at a core level. The potency of the mid-tide promotes health and healing in all tissues where it is able to manifest." (Kern, "Wisdom in the Body," 2005) Even though you may not be able to distinguish the difference between the surface (CRI), mid-tide, and deeper, slower long tide in your system, it will still benefit and respond to your conscious, intentional contact.

ONE SKY

The Cranial Sacral Hold

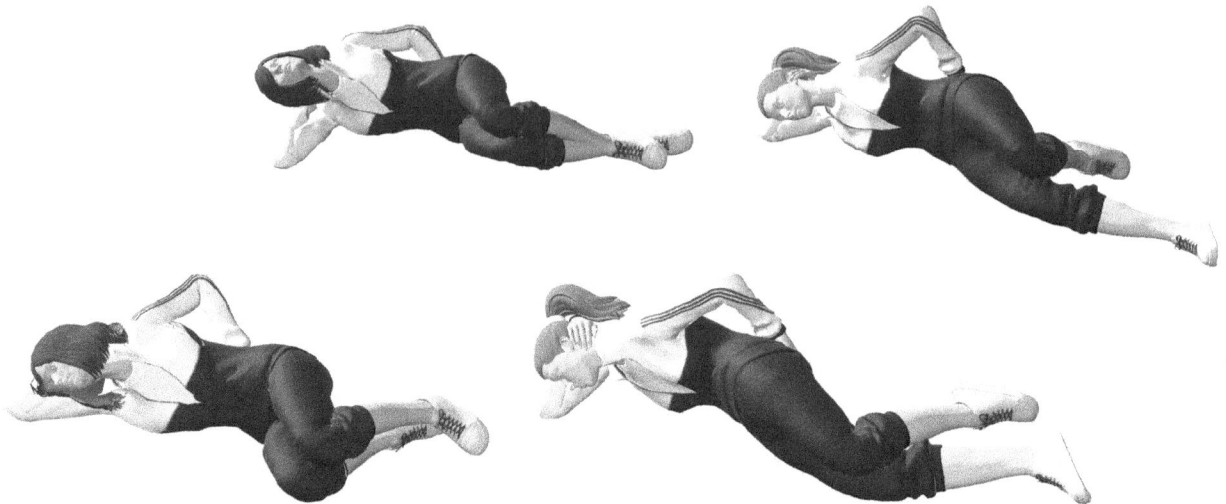

Group 1: Relax and hold

There is nothing to do for this self-treatment except to gently cradle the base of your skull while the other hand rests securely on your sacrum. Find the most comfortable position for both hands and shoulders, but forego it if your body can't get comfortable or if you have a shoulder injury.

One side might prove to be easier than the other in accepting the hand positions. There are a variety of options you can try, and you can stay there for several minutes or longer. Stay as long as you can, up to half an hour or more.

You can use this method to take the stress off at the end of the day to revitalize or to help sleep.

Groups 2 and 3: Sense, adjust, hold

Test for yourself the various hand, back, and leg positions that would increase the comfort level for your shoulder. You can also vary the angles that your head and neck are in to make it easier for the entire body to relax and sink into it.

There is no need to alter the breathing pattern on this exploration, but it may be good to notice if or how your breath changes as you maintain the hold. There may be a slight, rhythmic motion happening by itself between your hands. If you notice it, pay attention to whether the amplitude seems to increase and how that relates to your overall experience afterwards. Stay as long as you like.

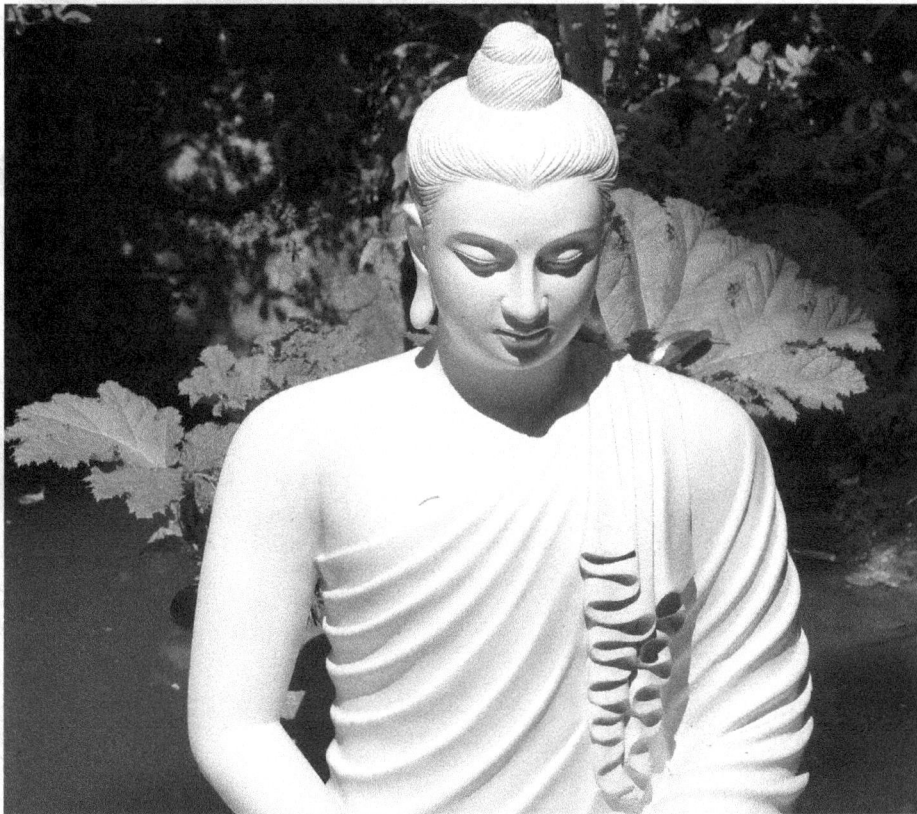

SECTION 6

Movements and Manual Therapy to Explore While Seated

> Sickness is an effect caused by the stoppage of some supply of fluid or quality of life... He conquers the disease by knowing how to apply the principles of this science along the lines of sensation, motion, and nutrition.
>
> A.T. Still, 1908

There is one brief chair sequence that has substantial value in all the ways it can benefit the time we spend seated. This last section will be for that sequence, along with a few manual self-treatments that can improve maneuverability while standing. Although you'll be in a different position, maintain as much as possible the intention of moving as a fluid, integrated whole.

The Wave

Group 1: Move your body as a unified whole

Use a chair that has room on the sides for your arms to move. First slide one hip forward-leading with the knee, then the other-like you were cross-country skiing. Repeat this motion a few times until you get into the rhythm of it.

Then arch your back gently as you let your arms swing back and forth in sync with the arching of your back and the rocking back and forth of your legs. Arch and swing the arms back, curl and bring the arms forward, even as far as crossing them in front of your body as you bend in the head, neck, and chest.

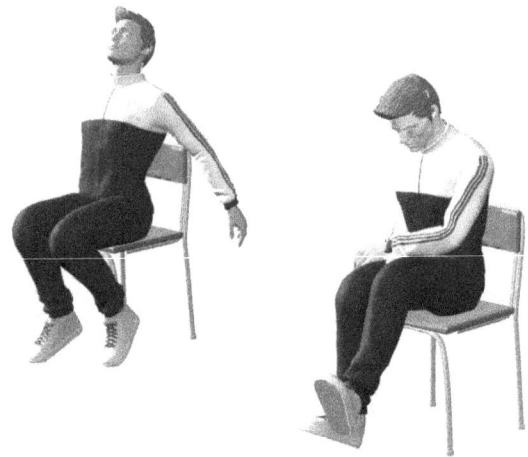

As an alternate option, you can lift one knee then the other when you curl and flex your upper body, rather than sliding the knees back and forth. You can also add flexing the foot to help extend the flexion all the way down the body to the feet.

Groups 2 and 3: Sense, breathe, listen, and move in harmony

Replicate the guidance for Group 1 but add an inhale as you arch, and an exhale as you flex your body. Explore how far and at which angle the arm swings should go in both directions to optimize the freedom in the midline.

Do the same for the slide and/or lift with your knee and notice what changes above and below your waist. You want to feel the releasing, but also the sensitizing (awakening) to your input, which enhances the smoothness and flow of the entire system.

Alternate with the external rotation of your arms (L-shaped) as you swing them behind you, then pivot the L in front like you're hugging yourself as you flex the body. Monitor your spine, sacrum, back, and shoulder muscles as you alternate positions, and notice which seems to be the most effective for your body that day.

Another possibility is to rotate your shoulders forward, up, around, and down as you swing the arms back, then rotate them the opposite direction as you flex. Experiment with turning your hips and feet outward as you arch, and inward as you flex. Whatever you choose, continue to prioritize making the motion smooth and effortless.

You can also explore adding the flexion and extension of your wrists and ankles to increase a fuller involvement of the tissue fields up through the arms and legs. Play with all of the possible combinations and listen to what your body thinks about them! Move slowly, be gentle.

Compare how this sequence works after sitting at a desk or at a meeting, or add it after exercising at the gym, gardening, or taking the dog out for a walk. In general, it's good to get a sense of which activities create tension in specific areas of your body, and which sequences work best for each scenario. This way you'll be able to reset your own system before things get away from you or accumulate into something that could lead to a more serious problem.

Freeing upstream transmission of force in the legs

The last exploration for the book will be one that, similar to the hand and wrist, can open restrictions in the ankle and foot (Fig. 6.8). Whether you've had a sprain or fracture, have high insteps and high arches, bunions, or flat feet, this manual therapy method will be helpful. At times, just the shoes we wear can bind the feet in such a way that their natural motion is impaired and becomes self-limiting. Hiking or work boots, high heels, sneakers that are laced all the way up, or any shoes that have pointy toes will put stress and strain on the feet and change the juxtaposition of the bones and connective tissue (Fig.6.7). They may become compressed and sticky. This could help unwind some of those factors.

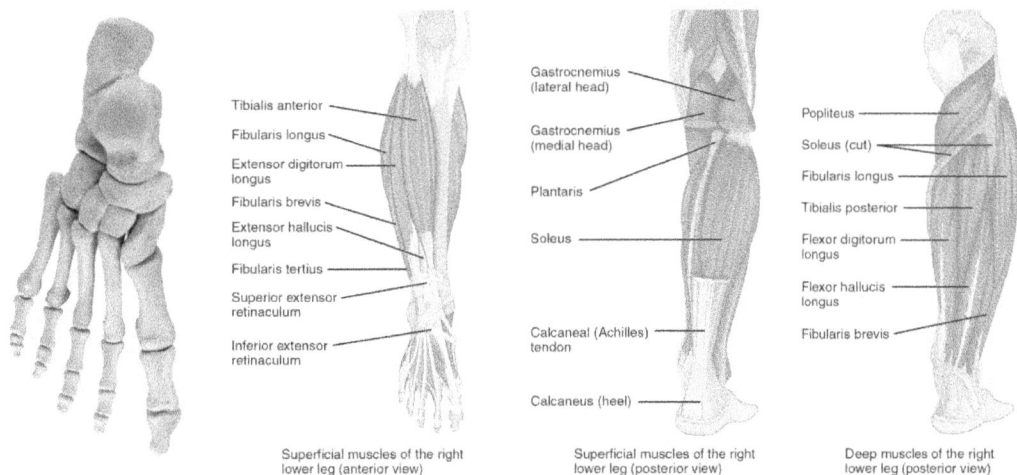

Fig. 6.7 – Bones of the feet

Fig. 6.8 – Muscles of the leg that move the feet with retinaculum of the ankle
Courtesy of OpenStax, CC BY 4.0, via Wikimedia Commons

ONE SKY

When the communication between the feet, ankles, and muscles that are intimately interconnected is uncompromised, everything you use them for will be more balanced, relaxed, and efficient, not to mention less painful. Countless times tension in the lower legs and thighs can be reduced if not resolved by aligning and decreasing intraosseous compression in the bones of the feet.

Opening the Gate

Group 1: Hold firmly, rotate, flex, and extend

Cross your legs with the ankle at or near the other knee. Take hold of the ankle with both hands and pull up on the surface layers of skin as you flex the foot up and back (dorsiflex and plantarflex).

Walk up the leg with your hands, keeping a firm grip and slight pull up toward the knee. Then wrap your hands around the ankle and twist both hands in one direction then the other as you flex the foot. If you can, repeat the twisting as you slowly rotate the foot.

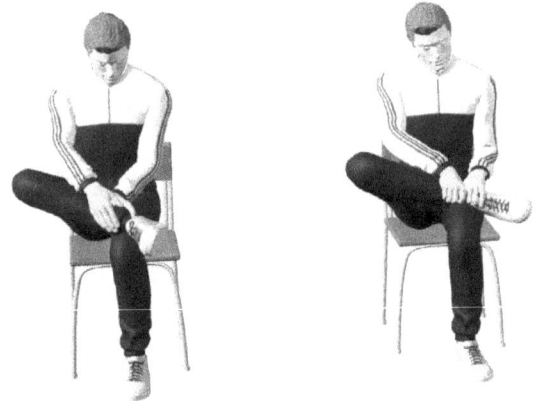

Don't twist too hard, but just enough to get hold of the surface skin and still be able to move the ankle freely. You want to loosen stickiness in the retinaculum over the tendons that pass through to the foot. Once is enough for this sequence, then change sides.

Groups 2 and 3: Sense, breathe, hold, adjust, and move

Follow the suggestions for Group 1 and see if inhaling and exhaling during dorsiflexion or plantar flexion increase responsiveness in the area. The movement of the foot itself promotes response to the contact input, so notice which rate and angle of motion elicits the best release. As an option, hold your hands steady while your rotate the foot as smoothly as you can.

You will find that taking care of the cumulative forces in the hands, wrists, ankles, and feet can do wonders for the arms, neck, legs, and hips. Relieving these restrictions from the extremities goes a long way toward creating ease and fluidity in the midline/core as well as in the joints, particularly the knees and elbows! They're also readily accessible so you don't have to go somewhere and lie down to be able to receive the benefit of these maneuvers. At your desk, watching television, or even at a meeting you can slip these little resets into your schedule and accomplish some helpful self-care that makes the rest of the day run more smoothly. Several meridians, nerves, and blood vessels also move through these tight regions, so you can get an energy boost along with the other benefits.

Similar to the ongoing need for food, rest, and water, movement and manual therapy are types of nourishment that the body needs on a regular basis. Just like anything else the body discharges that it doesn't need, leftover tensions should be discharged so the body can reset. It may not do it by itself as readily after a certain age, so it's really valuable to have your own set of resources to draw from to support the release and reorganization process so that it can rest and recharge more fully.

Freeing forces up through the arm using the hand and the joints

We used the Wall Press, Trees in the Wind, Tap Dance, and the Diaphragm sequences earlier to help open soft tissue up through the arm and connect the extremities to the midline and to one another. Those sequences were best experienced while standing or lying supine and side-lying. These next manual therapy methods to free the flow of information up through the arm are more suited to sitting, so the arm can rest on the leg or on the lap while you access the overworked areas.

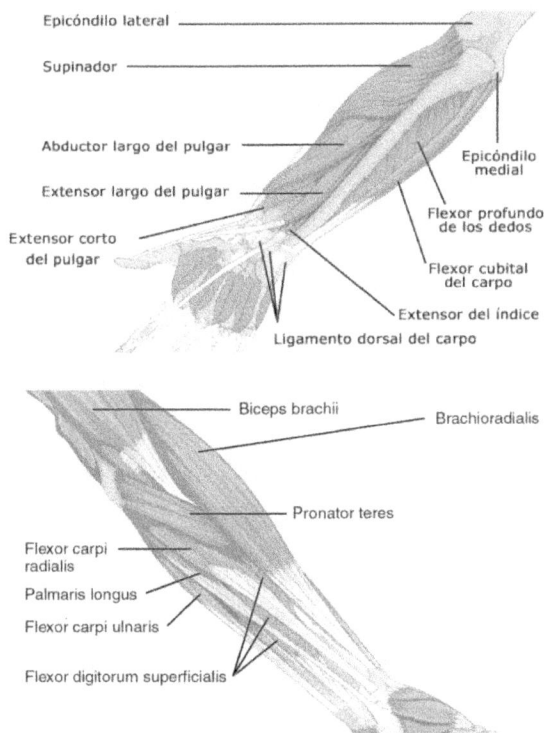

First, let's see what you'll be working with. We'll also be using the transformative power of the bones to communicate the changes we want to see up through the arm, all the while releasing the cumulative compressive forces and malalignments in sensitive joints spaces. We worked with the retinaculum a bit earlier around the wrist, which secures and protects the many tendons, nerves, and vessels that pass through that small area over the carpal bones. Now we'll work directly with the bones that are connected to the tendons, ligaments, and fascia that are intimately involved with muscle function.

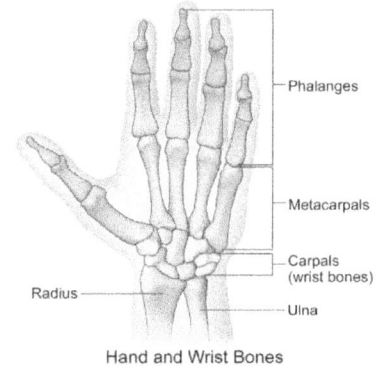

Figs. 6.11 and 6.12 - *Extensor and flexor muscles of the forearm that move the hand Courtesy of CFCF, CC BY-SA 4.0 via Wikimedia Commons*

Hand and Wrist Bones

Fig. 6.9 – Bones of the hand and wrist *Courtesy of Ceative Commons Attribution 3.0 Unported*

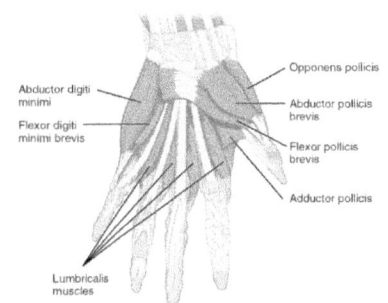

Fig. 6.10 – *Instrinsic muscles of the hand Courtesy of Creative Commons Attribution -Share Alike 4.0 International*

Opening the Tunnel

Initially, you'll be squeezing together the radius and ulna of the forearm by applying small amounts of pressure right at the area near the carpal bones (Fig. 6.9). You'll feel them as bony prominences that jut out to the side. The carpal bones, just beyond the radius and ulna in the direction of the hand, tend to become compressed with repetitive use patterns in fields like hairdressing, gardening, carpentry, computers, driving, painting, and those activities that require a lot of finger speed or dexterity. This sequence will be helpful for those types of overuse. Opening the Tunnel 2 using the fingers to release the muscles up the arm is also very helpful for the hands (Fig.6.10), which is the next sequence. It also supports the energy flow through the meridians, which are beneficial for many of the midline structures and general levels of tension in the soft tissue. These methods can also be applied to the bones of your ankles, feet, and toes.

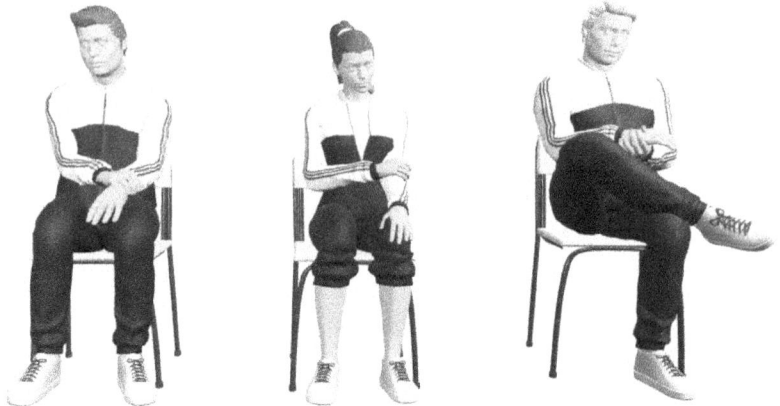

Opening the Tunnel 1

Group 1: Hold and squeeze

Hold your left wrist with your right hand where the bony prominences are on either side and gently squeeze in to the count of 5, and release slowly to the count of 8. Repeat 3 times.

Move to the carpal bones at the base of your hand and lightly press in, first from the sides, then from top to bottom of the hand. Squeeze slowly to the count of 4, and release to the count of 4. Repeat 3 times. Next, surround the bony prominences at the elbow (Fig.6.10) and slowly press them toward one another to the count of 3, and release to the count of 5. Repeat 3 times and switch sides.

Groups 2 and 3: Hold, sense, breathe

Follow the directions for Group 1, but sense whether your body is still opening after you are counting the bones back from being compressed. If they're still moving, let them come to rest before beginning the next compression. Explore different hand positions and angles for the compression, particularly if one side of the joint feels tighter than the other.

For example, when squeezing the epiphysis (end) of the ulnar and radius, you can try pressing slightly up toward the elbow at the same time you're squeezing in. In the same way, you can spread the carpal bones slightly away from one another as you press in from top to bottom.

ONE SKY

Opening the Tunnel 2

2-A 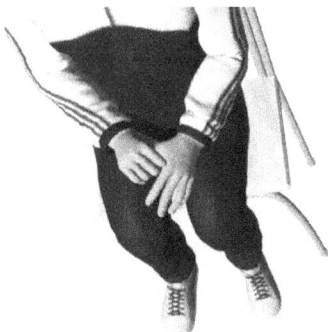 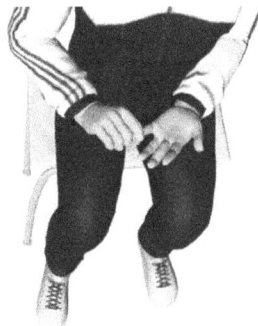 2-B

Group 1 (2-A): Hold, pull, and rotate

Sit so that both arms will be able to be relaxed. Wrap the working hand around the other thumb, resting along the vertical line of the bones in the thumb, or firmly around the base knuckle. (2-A) With a secure but gentle hold, pull it away from the wrist to the count of 4, and allow it to spring back to the count of 4. On the second go round, twist the thumb very slightly in one direction before you pull it and let it recoil. Then rotate it in the other direction slowly and gradually contain the recoil to the count of 4.

On the fourth round, pull it straight out at a slightly different angle, perhaps closer to or further away from the index finger. Repeat this process with each finger then switch sides. If you're in a rush, you can always just do this reset on the fingers that may be getting stiff or arthritic, but they each affect one another, so if you have time it's best to release them all.

Group 2 and 3 (2-A): Hold, listen, follow, and decompress

Use the general instructions for Group 1, and also notice whether, as you pull to decompress any finger (at the level of where the metacarpal bones meet the phalanges), it has a predisposed tendency to want to rotate in one direction or another. If you hold it lightly initially, it will more easily reveal its current preference. Once it shows itself, follow that tendency to the extent of its intrinsic torsion, then pull and hold it at the comfortable end range. The finger will begin to unwind and rotate itself back to center, whereupon you can then follow the recoil back into the joint and listen for any additional types of unwinding it may express there, in the hand, or up through the forearm (Figs. 6.11 and 6.12).

Allow it to continue until the forces have fully discharged. You can also decompress again and allow it to rock back and forth a bit more, or circumnavigate its relationship to the joint space. After this motion, when it recoils it will most likely be still and balanced.

If it's still moving, try visiting the other smaller joints in the finger and repeating the process. Attempt to slightly separate the articular surfaces of the joint and allow each bone to sway and unwind as you decompress the proximal (closer to the palm) from the more distal phalanges (Fig.6.9). As an alternative, you can add the compress/decompress of each knuckle approach in 2-B as you pull and rotate the joint capsules working your way up to the fingertips. Notice whether the muscles in your forearm or upper arm feel different after these sequences.

Group 1, 2, and 3 (2-B): Hold, press from sides and top/bottom

Taking one finger at a time, compress each knuckle from two directions to the count of 4, and release to the count of 4 twice. If the joint is painful, use less pressure. If done regularly, the pain will diminish or disappear.

The main takeaway here is that every part has a role to play in the whole. There are inherent intrinsic relationships that connect almost everything in the body, so it's always best to think of any part as a significant contributor to the well-being of the whole. Even if you can't feel it all the time during the day, it helps to know that your body has a vast subliminal life that is intentionally beneath your conscious perception most of the time. Once it reaches a certain threshold, the sensation or symptom will appear, but you're being encouraged to be proactive and attend to little imbalances before they become obvious bigger ones. Remember that soft tissue, fluid, energetic, and skeletal issues also influence the viscera, organs, glands, and nervous system, and vice-versa. So when you're taking care of anything, you're helping everything.

Most areas of the body and mind can also have a major influence upon the midline, including your hands, feet, fingers and toes, along with your beliefs, thoughts and emotions. The midline serves everything else, so keeping that open, supple, and awakened is a priority. Looking at the way you approach your work, exercise, or hobbies as a way to minimize the load on the midline is a supremely healthy perspective to use when organizing your activities and how you participate in them. Looking at the way you hold your perceptions and attitudes as well as your conflct resolution styles, is just as important as how you participate in an exercise routine.

Remember, these movement sequences are best viewed as guidance, suggestions, or recommendations, in addition to being supportive encouragement and inspiration. They're not set in stone; play with them! They are doors to perception that you can use to explore and discover the wants, needs, and preferences for your system's unwinding and reset. As was pointed out earlier in this Volume as well as in Volume 8, even your brain and internal organs will be supported and nourished by taking care of the midline. Some of you may remember the emphasis on the role the bones play in Volume 8, labeling them as a potential brain as well. For a truly fascinating exploration, try focusing on them as you reach, or rotate the long bones, and as you flex, or extend the spine. An entirely different world of responses that is even more global awaits.

There is more in the midline than just health and vitality, which are not minor attributes by any means. Once you've attuned to the ways that balance your inner qualities and systems, potentially you've also found your body's door to bliss. You're in your innernet. It's an invaluable reward in all of this: the life-long deepened relationship you gain with your own system. Once that door has been opened, it can remain available to you whether things are in or out of balance, and with your conscious input, offer insights into how to reestablish synchrony and open even more doors to inner peace, equanimity, and love.

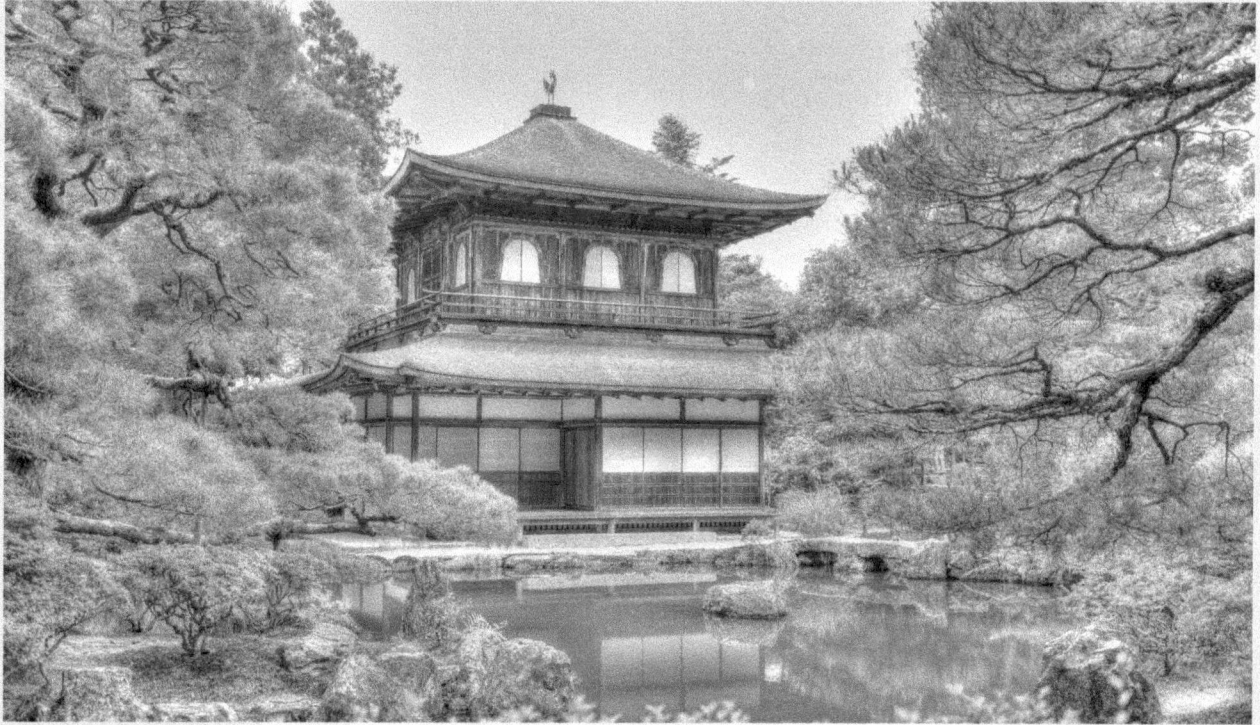

> "The dance is a poem of which each movement is a word."
>
> Mata Hari

References

1. Tian, et al., *"Heterogeneous aging across multiple organ systems and prediction of chronic disease and mortality,"* Nature Medicine; March, 2023

2. Chao Nie, et al., "Distinct biological ages of organs and systems identified from a multi- omics study, Cell Reports 38, March 8, 2022

3. vanBeek, Kirkwood and Bassingthwaighte, "Understanding the physiology of the ageing individual: computational modelling of changes in metabolism and endurance, Interface Focus, 2016

4. Drs. Meagan Wasfy, Adolph Hutter, and Rory Weiner,*"Sudden Cardiac Death in Athletes,"* Debakey-Journal XII (2) 2016

5. "Medical Research Studies NBA Players' Hearts," Black Health Matters.com, 2023)

6. UABMedicine, *"Basketball Players Suffer the Highest Rate of Sudden Cardiac Death,"* 2023

7. Brian Mossop, *"Death on the Basketball Court,"* The New Yorker, 2014

8. Semsarian, Ingles, and Wilde, *"Sudden cardiac death in the young: the molecular autopsy and a practical approach to surviving relatives,"* European Heart Journal (2105) 36, 1290- 1296

9. Michael Scott Emery, M.D. FACC; and Claudio Milstein, PhD, *"Dysfunctional Breathing in Athletes: A Brief Primer for the Sports Cardiologist,"* American College of Cardiology, May 11, 2022

10. *"Vitamin C: An Essential Nutrient for Good Lung and Respiratory Health,"* Respiratory Health, 19 March 2023

11. Yvette Brazier, *"Chinese exercise is good for the heart,"* Medical News Today, March 10, 2016

12. Lauren Bedosky, *"6 Potential Health Benefits of Qigong – A TCM Mind-Body Practice,"* Everyday Health, June 15, 2022

13. Michelle Fletcher, B.A., *"Strengthen the Heart with Qi Gong,"* Pacific College of Health and Science, 2023

14. Harvard Health Medical School, *"Mindfulness can improve heart health,"* February 1, 2018

15. Liu, et al, *"The Efficacy of Tai Chi and Qigong Exercises on Blood Levels of Nitric Oxide and Endothelin-1 in Patients with Essential Hypertension: a Systematic Review and Meta- Analysis of Randomized Controlled Trials,"* Evid. Based Complement Alternat Med 2020; 2020 Jul 30

16. Arjun Julka, "He had a Tai Chi master come to practice once": Kobe Bryant reveals the weirdest thing Phil Jackson made him do during practice," The Sports Rush, May 14, 2022

17. Lei Sun, MD, et al, *"Tai Chi can prevent cardiovascular disease and improve cardiopulmonary function of adults with obesity aged 50 years and older,"* Medicine, 2019 Oct; 98(42)

18. Carolyn Gregoire, *"Yoga and Meditation Shown to Drastically Reduce Hospital Visits,"* Science, October 28, 2016

19. Lima, Martins, and Reed, *"Physiological Responses Induced by Manual Therapy in Animal Models: a Scoping Review,"* Frontiers in Neuroscience, 08 May 2020

20. Tori Hudson, ND, *"Hibiscus, Hawthorne, and the Heart,"* Natural Medicine Journal, March 22, 2014

21. Jie Wang, Xingjjang Xiong, Bo Feng, *"Effect of Crataegus in Cardiovascular Disease Prevention: an Evidence-Based Study,"* Evidence Based Complementary and Alternative Medicine, November, 2013

22. Jin Dai and Russell J. Mumper, *"Plant Phenolics: Extraction, analysis and Their Antioxidant and Anticancer Properties,"* Molecules, 2010 Oct; 15(10) 7313-7352

23. Lin Jin, et.al, *"Gallic acid improves cardiac dysfunction and fibrosis in pressure overload- induced heart failure,"* Scientific Reports, 18 June 2018

24. Somya Binu, MSc., *"Arjuna: This Herbal Hero Protects Your Heart Health,"* netmeds.com, September 13. 2021

25. Dr. Vikram Chauhan, *"Arjuna – Best Herb for Heart Care,"* Planet Ayurveda, August 8, 2023

26. Eftychia Kotronia, et al, *"Oral health and all-cause cardiovascular disease, and respiratory mortality in older people in the UK and USA,"* Scientific Reports, 2021

27. Robert H. Shmerling, MD, *"Gum disease and the connection to heart disease,"* Harvard Health Publishing, April 22, 2021

28. Lu Han, et al., *"Single cell transcriptomics identifies a signaling network coordinating endoderm and mesoderm diversification during foregut organogenesis,"* Nature Communications, 2020

29. Bruno Bordoni, Navid Mahabadi, Matthew Varacello, "Anatomy, Fascia," National Library of Medicine, 2023 Jul 17

30. Han, et al., *"Changes in nuclear pore numbers control nuclear import and stress response of mouse hearts,"* Developmental Cell, Vol. 67, Issue 20, P2397-2411, October 24, 2022

31. Alisson C. Cardoso, et al., *"Mitochondrial substrate utilization regulates cardiomyocyte cell-cycle progression,"* Nature Metabolism, Vol. 2 February 2020, 167-178

32. Ana Catarina Silva, et al., *"Bearing My Heart: The Role of Extracellular Matrix on Cardiac Development, Homeostasis, and Injury Response,"* Frontiers in Cell and Developmental Biology, 12 January 2021

33. Gondalia, et. al, *"Cardiac Plasticity in Health and Disease,"* Translational Cardiology, January, 2012

34. Watson, Perbellini, and Terracciano, *"Cardiac t-tubules: where structural plasticity meets functional adaptation",* Cardiovascular Research (2016) 112, 423-425

35. Gregory Lim, *"Complexity and plasticity of cardiac cellular composition,"* Cell Biology, Nature Reviews/ Cardiology, Volume 17, December 2020

36. *Fotius G. Pitoulis and Cesare M. Terracciano, "Heart Plasticity in Response to Pressure and Volume-Overload. A Review of Findings in Compensated and Decompensated Phenotypes,"* Frontiers in Physiology, 13 February 2020

37. Troy James Cross, Chui-Ho Kim, Bruce D. Johnson, and Sophie Lalande, *"The interactions between respiratory and cardiovascular systems in systolic heart failure,"* Journal of Applied Physiology, 128: 214-224, 2020

38. Katherine Ka-Yin Yau and Alice Yuen Loke, *"Effects of diaphragmatic deep breathing exercises for prehypertensive or hypertensive adults: A literature review,"* Complement. Ther. Clin. Pract., 2021 May

39. Rachael Lowe, *"Muscles of Respiration,"* Physiopedia, 2023

40. Pilar Gerasimo, *"Emotional Biochemistry",* Experience Life, Brain Health/Functional/ Integrative Medicine, November 2020

41. Nummenmaa and Touminen, *"Opioid system and human emotions,"* British Journal of Pharmacology, 175(14), 2017

42. Paul Govern, *"Study finds aerobic exercise spurs endorphins, relieves low back pain,"* Vanderbilt University Medical Center Reporter, August 5, 2020

43. Paula Boaventura, Sónia Jaconiano, and Filipa Ribero, *"Yoga and Qigong for Health: Two Sides of the Same Coin?"* Behavioral Sciences, 2022 July; 12(7) 222

44. Dipak Hemraj and Dr. Lewis Jassey, *"What is 2-Arachidonoylyglyerol?,"* Leafwell, 2023

45. A. Dietrich and W. F. McDaniel, *"Endocannabinoids and exercise,"* Br J Sports Med 2004;38:536-541

46. Michael Siebers, et al., *"Exercise-induced euphoria and anxiolysis (sedation) do not depend on endogenous opioids in humans,"* Psychoneuroendocrin., Vol. 126, April 2021

47. Alexandros Serianos, et al., *"The Role of Physical Exercise in Opioid Substitution Therapy: Mechanisms of Sequential Effects,"* IJMS, 21 February 2023

48. Sigrid Breit, et al., *"Vagus Nerve as Modulator of the Brain-Gut Axis in Psychiatric and Inflammatory Disorders,"* Fronteirs in Psychiatry, March 2018

49. Hashim, Albayanti, and Nazal, *"Heart Memory and Feelings,"* Heart Transplantation, 12 January 2023

50. Madure,*"Neurocardiology: The Brain in the Heart"*, June 15, 2008

51. Alshami, *"Pain: Is It All in the Brain or the Heart,"* Current Pain Headache Report, 2019 November 14; 23(12):88

52. Professor Mohammed Omar Salem, *"The Heart, Mind, and Sprit,"* 2007

53. Lynne Eldrige, MD, *"What is the Thymus Gland – Playing a role in immunity, autoimmunity, and aging,"* VeryWell Healthy, July 11, 2023

54. Camilla Ciapponi, et al., Frontiers in Systems Neuroscience, 10 May 2023

55. Cleveland Clinic, "The But-Grain Connection," 2023

56. Carabotti, et al, "The gut-brain axis: interactions between enteric microbiota, central *and enteric nervous systems,"* Annals of G   astroenterology," 2015 Apr-June; 28(2): 203-208

57. Jenkins and Lumpkin, *"Developing a sense of touch,"* Development, 2017 Nov 15; 144(22): 4078-4090

58. Casey Henley, Foundations of Neuroscience, 2021

A special thanks to Wikimedia Commons, Creative commons, Pexels and Pixabay for providing access to many images in this text.

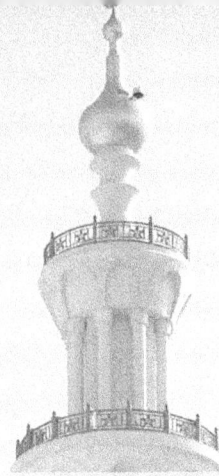

"*From the collection of the pieces, it is evident, that when we separate from our Health at an early age, one part of the embryo stays around us like a guardian angel, and does not return inside until we fall in love with the Health, recognizing it as our true self. Then we are safe from self- destruction and self-betrayal.*"

Dr. James Jealous, An Osteopathic Odyssey

Image courtesy of Pavlo Luchkovski and Pexels

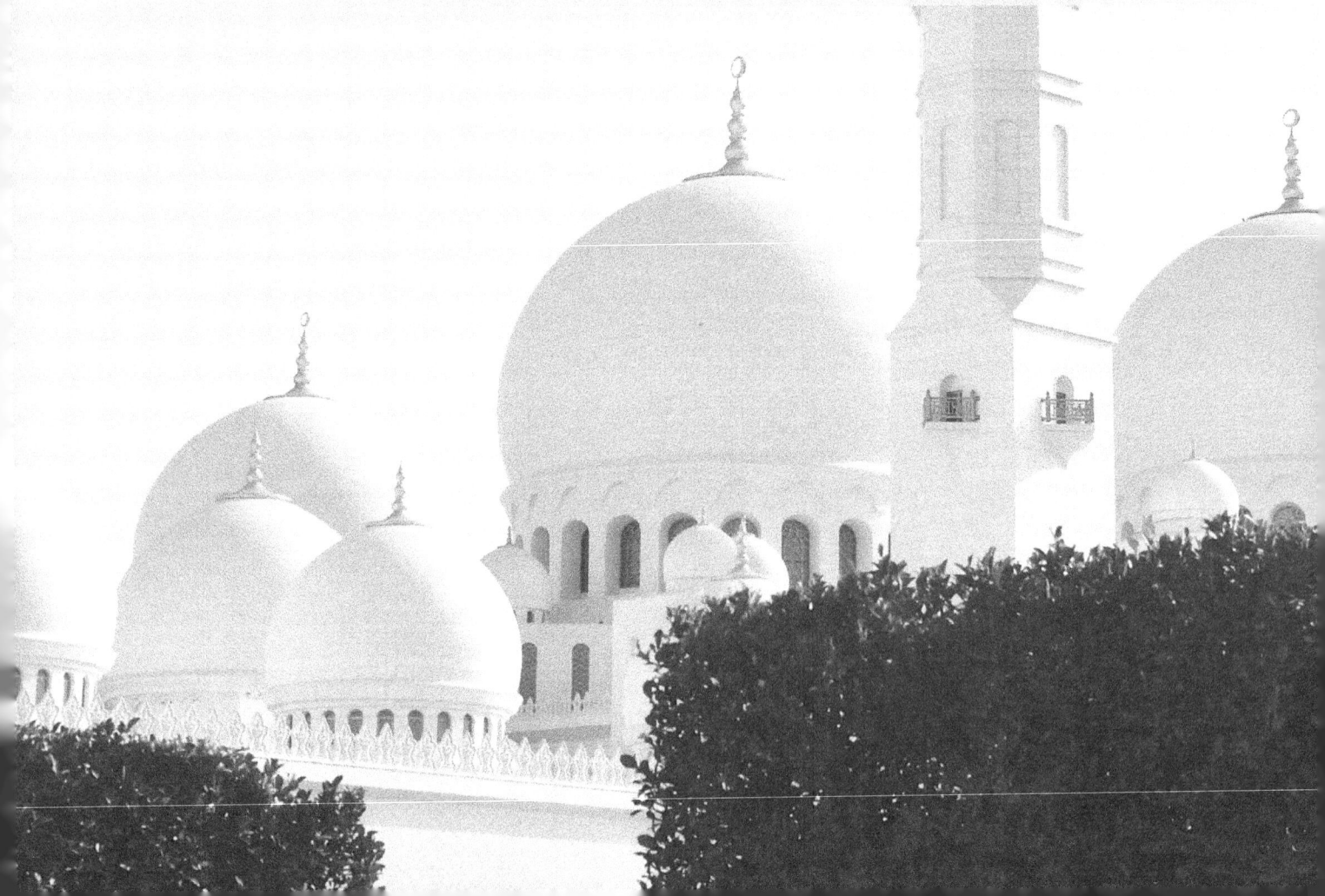